Antibiotic Resistance
A Threat to World Health
A Selected Annotated Bibliography
on
Bacteria, Viruses, Fungi, and other Pathogens
and a Complete Copy of the CDC Report
Antibiotic Resistance
Threats in the United States, 2013

H. G. Brack, Editor
Judy Weed, Assistant Editor
Davistown Museum
Department of Environmental History

Phenomenology of Biocatastrophe
Publication Series Volume 4

ISBN 13: 978-1533029997

This publication is sponsored by

Davistown Museum

Department of Environmental History

www.davistownmuseum.org

and

Engine Company No. 9

Radscan-Chemfall
Est. 1970

Disclaimer

Engine Company No. 9 relocated to Maine in 1970. The staff members of Engine Company No. 9 are not members of, affiliated with, or in contact with, any municipal or community fire department in the State of Maine.

Comments, criticisms, and suggestions are welcomed and may be directed to:
curator@davistownmuseum.org

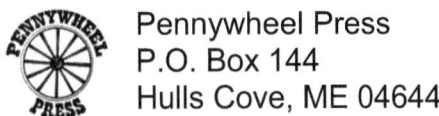

Pennywheel Press
P.O. Box 144
Hulls Cove, ME 04644

1985-2000 Publications Sponsored by Engine Company No. 9
Station 4, Hulls Cove, ME
and
The Center for Biological Monitoring

Radscan: Information Sampler on Long-Lived Radionuclides: 1990-1999

A Review of Radiological Surveillance Reports of Waste Effluents in Marine Pathways at the Maine Yankee Atomic Power Company at Wiscasset, Maine--- 1970-1984: An Annotated Bibliography

Legacy for Our Children: The Unfunded Costs of Decommissioning the Maine Yankee Atomic Power Station: The Failure to Fund Nuclear Waste Storage and Disposal at the Maine Yankee Atomic Power Station: A Commentary on Violations of the 1982 Nuclear Waste Policy Act and the General Requirements of the Nuclear Regulatory Commission for Decommissioning Nuclear Facilities

Patterns of Noncompliance: The Nuclear Regulatory Commission and the Maine Yankee Atomic Power Company: Generic and Site-Specific Deficiencies in Radiological Surveillance Programs

RADNET: Nuclear Information on the Internet: General Introduction; Definitions and Conversion Factors; Biologically Significant Radionuclides; Radiation Protection Guidelines

RADNET: Anthropogenic Radioactivity: Plume Pulse Pathways, Baseline Data and Dietary Intake

RADNET: Anthropogenic Radioactivity: Chernobyl Fallout Data: 1986 – 2001

RADNET: Anthropogenic Radioactivity: Major Plume Source Points

Integrated Data Base for 1992: U.S. Spent Fuel and Radioactive Waste Inventories, Projections, and Characteristics: Reprinted from October 1992 Oak Ridge National Laboratory Report DOE/RW-0006, Rev 8

2000-2015 Publications Sponsored by
Davistown Museum Department of Environmental History
and Engine Company No. 9, Station 4, Hulls Cove, ME

Essays on Biocatastrophe and the Collapse of Global Consumer Society. Vol. 1. 2010.

Biocatastrophe Lexicon: An Epigrammatic Journey Through the Tragedy of our Round-World Commons. Vol. 2. 2010.

Biocatastrophe: The Legacy of Human Ecology: Toxins, Health Effects, Links, Appendices, and Bibliographies. Vol. 3. 2010.

Antibiotic Resistance: A Threat to World Health: A Selected Annotated Bibliography on Bacteria, Viruses, Fungi, and other Pathogens and a Complete Copy of the CDC Report Antibiotic Resistance Threats in the United States, 2013. Vol. 4. 2016.

Where Have All the Plastics Gone? Ménage à Trois in the Sea Surface Microlayer: Nanoparticles as Vectors of Environmental Chemicals. Vol. 5. 2015.

Table of Contents

Preface

The mission of Volume 4 of the Phenomenology of Biocatastrophe publication series is to provide timely commentary and updates on the emergence and growth of antibiotic resistant and viral infections, as well as on other important widespread threats to human health such as the Zika outbreak, Legionnaire's disease, norovirus infections, and the rapid increase in Lyme disease. There is a broad spectrum of antibiotic resistant microbes (ARM) now impacting a wide variety of bacteria, fungi, pathogens, and other microbial communities. The venues for their identification are the same hospitals, clinics, and research laboratories that lead to the pioneering adaptation of antimicrobial organisms to fight infectious diseases in developed and developing nations. In the United States, the CDC (Center for Disease Control) is the most important source of information on acquired bacterial resistance in human health, including its proliferation in the general community. The CDC publication, *Antibiotic Resistance: Threats in the United States, 2013* is reprinted in its entirety in Appendix 1 of this text.

An annotated selection of some of the most important NGO and international governmental (e.g. WHO) research on emerging bacterial infections and their sources precede the CDC 2013 report. The bibliographies are introduced by an overview of the historical context of the growth of antibiotic resistant microbes, including those in ancient microbiomes of the distant past, and a synopsis of other infections of interest. Commentary includes observations about the human biome and the environmental, economic, social, and public health sources of resistant bacteria now rapidly spreading throughout the health care systems of the world and the communities they serve.

The United States and other developed nations have sophisticated public health systems that can quickly identify and then, at least partially, mitigate the impact of antibiotic resistant diseases (ABRD). In other countries, a much smaller percentage of the population has access to the sophisticated medical facilities that characterize developed nations. In vulnerable BRIC (Brazil, Russia, India, China) nations of the developing world, hundreds of millions, if not billions, of citizens do not have access to clean water supplies or adequate sewage systems. The impact of antibiotic resistant diseases increases as the population within any nation lacks access to potable water or sophisticated public health services. The reality of health care inequality (synonymous with fresh water inequality) also affects many US citizens, as shown by the recent outbreak of Legionnaire's disease in Flint, MI, with its high levels of lead in its drinking water.

The potential impact of pandemics derived from a wide variety of microorganisms pose increasing public health threats as world population and frequency of international travel increase, factors supplementing the rising threat of antibiotic resistant diseases.

The threat of antibiotic resistance is now worldwide. Our global world community is now, in effect, getting smaller just as its supplies of potable fresh water, including fossil water, are being rapidly depleted, a topic to be further explored in volume 6 of this publication series. The growing world water crisis includes ever-growing quantities of bacterial and chemical contaminants, depletion of surface and underground potable water by consumption that exceeds replenishment, desertification, and flooding events that effectively transport contaminants to all water supplies. This is the hemispheric water cycle context for the growing spread of antibiotic resistant microbes within the human biome. Overpopulation, warfare, income inequality, lack of public resources, and ongoing infrastructure collapse all make their contributions to the proliferation of antibiotic resistance in both health care and community environments.

Introduction

The fundamental question about antibiotic resistant diseases (ABRD) is where and when did they originate? The answer lies in that huge panorama of microbiomes that are the basis for life on Earth. This vast landscape, which includes all aquatic and terrestrial environments, has its roots in ancient bacterial communities that can be traced back billions of years. Many now lost microbes once inhabited ancient bacterial microbiomes in all trophic levels of the biosphere. Their descendents continue to live in all the microbiomes that characterize the biosphere, one of hundreds of millions of which is the human gut. Human intestines are characterized by as many as 100 trillion microorganisms belonging to 200 or more microbial species. Thousands of years before the development of industrial agriculture and before the evolution of hospital-acquired infections, ancient environmental reservoirs of resistance characterized all microbiomes, including the microbial communities characterizing the human gut (stomach and intestines), skin, the vaginal environment, the lungs and nose and the oral environment of the mouth. A number of annotated citations in this text discuss these ancient reservoirs of bacteria and the change in the genes that evolved to counteract or control other bacterial infections.

A whole new world of manmade environmental chemicals now characterizes our hemispheric water cycle, including all biomes, whose key constituent is water. Only a small percentage of the total volume of these effluents can be biodegraded or bioconverted to other metabolites by the many microbial communities in our round world commons. Water cycle contaminants range from persistent organic pollutants (POPs) to the many shorter lived environmental chemicals, many of which are the byproducts of the Age of Plastics, Information Technology, and Nanotechnology. Our many chemical effluents are the downside of a constantly growing global consumer society, which now includes the invisible threat of the spread of antibiotic resistance. Highly visible social crises such as the growing refuge populations in Europe, are characteristic of a world in political crisis. The evolution of microbial communities, which cannot be controlled by human technology, occurs outside of the limelight of social, political, or electronic media. The many battles of the microbes may become the most important form of warfare in the late Anthropocene.

The rapidly changing microbial communities of our contemporary medical and community health care systems highlighted by the CDC report on ABRD are part of a much larger worldwide panorama of viral infections such as HIV, malaria, cholera, influenza, and rabies. Many of these pandemics have been halted by the vaccines produced by the world medical community. Polio and smallpox head the list of dangerous plagues that are now medical history. Ebola has recently been controlled.

The impact of SARS has been curtailed. The Zika outbreak is now the object of a mass research effort to find a vaccine. Other emerging viral infections pose a future threat of worldwide pandemics. New variations of avian and livestock influenza, SARS, the Marburg virus, and other infections are now much more susceptible to hemispheric transport, sometimes associated with the increasing frequency of invasive species movement. The rapid spread of Lyme disease is an example of a viral infection that, unlike bacterial infections, cannot be treated with antibiotics, even if such treatments are used frequently. All bacterial and viral infections are occurring in the context of a rapidly growing world population and an expanding global consumer society. Contemporary society is now characterized by growing income inequality and a dramatic lack of funding for basic infrastructure maintenance. The presence of many challenges presented by the growth of antibiotic bacteria combines with growing political paralysis, at least in the United States, and a lack of informed consensus, all of which encourages the growing health care inequality that the world population now faces. Despite a dedicated and innovative med-techno-elite, the reality of the ecological impact of our beloved petrochemical-industrial-consumer product culture is the unfortunate downside of the glowing florescence of humanity in the Anthropocene. The phenomenon of antibiotic resistance is a hidden footnote to the gradual contamination and depletion of a vulnerable finite world water cycle. The many links between the imposition of human ecology on natural ecological systems and the evolution of antibiotic resistance microbes (ARMs) will long remain a subject for future research and documentation.

News Bites

The following selection of quotations provide an overview of the subject matter of this publication. Martin Blaser's 2015 publication *Missing Microbes: How the Overuse of Antibiotics is Fueling our Modern Plague*, a particularly comprehensive overview of the threat of antibiotic resistance, helps define the many historical and contemporary ramifications of both the lack of effective antibiotics and the impact of antibiotic resistance.

"Antibiotic therapy, if indiscriminately used, may turn out to be a medicinal flood that temporarily cleans and heals, but ultimately destroys life itself." (Felix Marti-Ibanez 1995)

"30 percent to 50 percent of antibiotics prescribed in hospitals are unnecessary or incorrect." (CDC 2013)

"Sediments of aquaculture farms are important antibiotic resistance regions where various antimicrobials and ARGs are concentrated." (Zhang 2009)

"As many other chemical pollutants, for example, persistent organic pollutants and heavy metals, ARGs are well-known "easy-to-get, hard-to-lose" pollutants." (Zhang 2009)

"There is regrowth of bacteria in drinking water distribution systems." (Xi 2009)

"Between 1997 and 2008, the percentage of children with diagnosed peanut allergy more than tripled." (Blaser 2015)

"Macro lead use is highest in the states with the highest obesity." (Blaser 2015)

"Today, about 1 in 88 children has autism or an autism-spectrum disorder (ASD)." (Blaser 2015)

"The 'disappearing microbiome hypothesis'…99% of all bacteria are killed by factors found in blood." (Blaser 2015)

"Loss of friendly gut bacteria at this early stage of development is driving obesity, at least in mice." (Blaser 2015)

"Invisible microbes comprise the sheer bulk of the Earth's biomass." (Blaser 2015)

"At least 20 million types of marine microbes (possibly 1 billion) make up 50 to 90% of the ocean's biomass." (Blaser 2015)

"Your body is composed of an estimated 30 trillion human cells, but it is host to more than 100 trillion bacterial and fungal cells." (Blaser 2015)

"Smell is important and it is mostly microbial in origin." (Blaser 2015)

"The average American child received nearly three courses of antibiotics in his or her first two years of life." (Blaser 2015)

"All mixed populations of bacteria include both susceptible and resistant bacteria." (Blaser 2015)

"When susceptible species are diminished or killed, populations of resistant bacteria expand. With fewer competitors around, resistant bacteria flourish." (Blaser 2015)

"About 40% of women in the United States today get antibiotics during delivery, which means some 40% of newborn infants are exposed to drugs just as they are acquiring their microbes." (Blaser 2015)

"New diseases related to the loss of *H. pylori* are rising." (Blaser 2015)

"Esophageal adenocarcinoma now has the fastest rising incidence of all major cancers, a six-fold increase in the last three decades." (Blaser 2015)

"Each of us has an army of memory cells, most of which remember some chemical aspect of a particular event, such as a component of a bacterial wall from a prior infection." (Blaser 2015)

"In 2011 a group of Dutch investigators reported on their examination of pharmacy records for all 577,627 children born in Denmark as singletons (not twins) between 1995 and 2003. Those who developed early IBD (inflammatory bowel disease) were 84% more likely to have received antibiotics. Furthermore, children who had taken antibiotics had more than triple the risk of developing Crohn's disease than those who were antibiotic-free. The more often they took antibiotics, the higher the risk." (Blaser 2015)

"A Canadian study…showed double the risk of asthma in children who received antibiotics in the first year of life. The prevalence of both hay fever and eczema has been rising dramatically in recent years paralleling the increase in asthma." (Blaser 2015)

"Virtually all antibacterial agents exert similar effects promoting growth on farm animals; the animals get bigger whether they receive penicillins, tetracyclines, or macrolides…all antibiotics produce more or less equivalent harmful collateral effects on our human resident bacteria." (Blaser 2015)

"The fate…of that estrogen molecule in the intestine depends on whether it meets a microbe that uses it as a meal or not." (Blaser 2015)

"With a huge world population that is essentially contiguous, and with so many of us with weakened defenses because of our compromised internal ecosystems, we are vulnerable as never before." (Blaser 2015)

"Global warming may not be our biggest worry…When the plague comes, it could be fast and intense." (Blaser 2015)

"Antibiotic use in China is even higher than it is in the United States." (Blaser 2015)

"C. diff. can wreak terrible damage when competing bacteria are wiped out by antibiotics…Hospitals are dangerous places – C. diff. has escaped the confines of the hospital and is now loose within the community." (Blaser 2015)

"In the United States, at least 250,000 people are hospitalized each year for C. diff. infections that they acquired there or at home, and 14,000 die as a result." (Blaser 2015)

"Globally, 5% of TB cases were estimated to have had multidrug-resistant TB (MDR-TB) in 2014. Drug resistance surveillance data show that an estimated 480,000 people developed MDR-TB in 2014 and 190,000 people died as a result of MDR-TB. Extensively drug-resistant TB (XDR-TB) has been reported by 105 Countries in 2014. On average, an estimated 9.7% of people with MDR-TB have XDR-TB." (World Health Organization 2015b)

Links

Alliance for the Prudent Use of Antibiotics (APUA) -- http://www.tufts.edu/med/apua/

Center for Disease Dynamics, Economics and Policy (CDDEP) -- http://www.cddep.org/

European Antimicrobial Resistance Surveillance System -- http://www.earss.rivm.nl

European Center for Ecotoxicology and Toxicology -- www.ecetoc.org www.exetocetoxmodels.org

GISP: Gonococcal Isolate Surveillance Project -- http://www.cdc.gov/std/gisp/default.htm

Human Microbiome Project at NYU -- http://gerd.med.nyu.edu/hmp

Infectious Diseases Society of America -- http://www.idsociety.org/Index.aspx

International census of marine microbes -- http://icomm.mbl.edu/

National Antimicrobial Resistance Monitoring System for Enteric Bacteria -- http://www.cdc.gov/narms/

National Healthcare Safety Network -- http://www.cdc.gov/nhsn/

Natural Resources Defense Council: Health Documents -- http://docs.nrdc.org/health/

NG-MAST: Neisseria gonorrhoeae multi antigen sequence typing -- www.ng-mast.net

RxList: The Internet Drug Index: http://www.rxlist.com/script/main/hp.asp

Acronyms

AGP	Antimicrobial growth promoter
API	Active pharmaceutical ingredient
ARB	Antibiotic-resistant bacteria
ARPA-E	Advanced Research Projects Agency - Energy
ASD	Autism spectrum disorder
C. diff	Clostridium difficile
CAFO	Concentrated animal feeding operations
CA-MRSA	Community-acquired methicillin-resistant Staphylococcus aureus
CDC	Centers for Disease Control and Prevention
DDD	Defined daily dose
DES	Diethylstilbestrol
EARSS	European antimicrobial resistance surveillance system
EI	Emerging infection
EID	Emerging infectious disease
ERA	Environmental risk assessment
ESBL	Extended-spectrum beta-lactamase
FMT	Fecal microbiota transplantation
GERD	Gastro esophageal reflux disease
GISP	Gonococcal Isolate Surveillance Project
HPV	Human papilloma virus
HACCP	Hazard analysis and critical control point
HA-MRSA	Hospital-acquired methicillin-resistant Staphylococcus aureus
HPC	Heterotrophic plate count
IBD	Inflammatory bowel disease
ICARE	Intensive care antimicrobial resistance epidemiology

IDSA	The Infectious Diseases Society of America
IFPRI	International Food Policy Research Institute
ISRAR	International surveillance of reservoirs of antibiotic resistance
LAB	Lactic acid bacteria
LTCF	Long-term care facility
MDR	Multidrug resistance
MDR-TB	Multidrug-resistant tuberculosis
MDRGN	Multidrug-resistant gram-negative organism
MNP	Metal nanoparticle
MRSA	Methicillin-resistant Staphylococcus aureus
MSSA	Methicillin-sensitive Staphylococcus aureus
NARMS	National antimicrobial resistance monitoring system
NICU	Neonatal intensive care unit
OCP	Organochlorine pesticide
PAT	Pulsed antibiotic treatment
PCR	Polymerase chain reaction
PhAC	Pharmaceutically active compound
SARS	Severe acute respiratory syndrome
SSAR	Sewage sludge antibiotic residue
STP	Sewage treatment plant
UK	United Kingdom
VLBW	Very low birth weight
VRE	Vancomycin-resistant Enterococci

Bibliography

Aarestrup, F., Bager, F. and Andersen, J. (2000). Association between the use of avilamycin for growth promotion and the occurrence of resistance among Enterococcus faecium fron broilers; epidemiological study and changes over time. *Microbial Drug Resistance*. 6L. pg. 71-5. http://www.ncbi.nlm.nih.gov/pubmed/10868810

Aarestrup, F. (2005). Veterinary drug usage and antimicrobial resistance in bacteria of animal origin. *Basic & Clinical Pharmacology & Toxicology*. 96. pg. 271-81. http://onlinelibrary.wiley.com/doi/10.1111/j.1742-7843.2005.pto960401.x/abstract

- "In Denmark it has been possible to reduce the usage of antimicrobial agents for food animals significantly and in general decreases in resistance have followed."

Abeylath, S. C., Turos, E., Dickey, S. and Lim, D. (2008). Glyconanobiotics: Novel carbohydrated nanoparticle antibiotics for MRSA and *Bacillus anthracis*. *Bioorganic & Medicinal Chemistry*. 16. pg. 2412-18. http://biology.usf.edu/cmmb/abl/data/Abeylath-Lim-2008-BMC.pdf

Abrahams, Peter. (2009). *120 Diseases*. Amber Books, London, England.

Abutaleb, Y., McNeill, R. and Nelson, D. J. (September 7, 2016). A most unwanted list. *Reuters*. http://www.reuters.com/investigates/special-report/usa-uncounted-cdc/

Adams, C., Wang, Y., Lofton, K. and Meyer, M. (2002). Removal of antibiotics from surface and distilled water in conventional water treatment processes. *Journal of Environmental Engineering*. 128(3). pg. 253-60. https://pubs.er.usgs.gov/publication/70024787

Aiello, A. (2003). Antibacterial cleaning and hygiene products as an emerging risk factor for antibiotic resistance in the community. *The Lancet Infectious Diseases*. 3(4). http://www.ncbi.nlm.nih.gov/pubmed/12901892

- "In recent years, there has been a proliferation of household products containing antibacterial agents such as triclosan (2,4,4' –trichloro-2'-hydroxyphenly ether) has been raised since it has been suggested that these products may contribute to resistance…Used for cleaning and disinfection within the home environment."

Alexanter, T., et al. (2008). Effect of subtherapeutic administration of antibiotics on the prevalence of antibiotic-resistant Escherichia coli bacteria in feedlot cattle. *Applied and Environmental Microbiology*. pg. 4405-16. http://aem.asm.org/content/74/14/4405.abstract

- "Antibiotic-resistant *Escherichia coli* in 300 feedlot steers receiving subtherapeutic levels of antibiotics was investigated through the collection of

3,300 fecal samples over a 314-day period. Antibiotics were selected based on the commonality of use in the industry and included chlortetracycline plus sulfamethazine (TET-SUL), chlortetracycline (TET), virginiamycin, monensin, tylosin or no antibiotic supplementation (control).Steers were initially fed a barley silage-based diet, followed by transition to a barley grain-based diet."

- "Irrespective of treatment, the prevalence of steers shedding TET-resistant *E. coli* was higher in animals fed grain-based compared to silage-based diets."
- "Subtherapeutic administration of tetracycline in combination with sulfamethazine increased the prevalence of tetracycline-and AMP-resistant *E. coli* in cattle. However, resistance to antibiotics may be related to additional environmental factors such as diet."

Allen, H. K., Donato, J., Wang, H. W., et al. (2010). Call of the wild: antibiotic resistance genes in natural environments. *Nature Reviews Microbology*. Vol. 8. pg. 251-259. http://www.nature.com/nrmicro/journal/v8/n4/abs/nrmicro2312.html

- "Environmental reservoirs of resistance determinants are poorly understood…This Review explores the presence and spread of antibiotic resistance in non-agricultural, non-clinical environments and demonstrates the need for more intensive investigation on this subject."
- "Some organisms and some environments harbor antibiotic resistance genes irrespective of the human use of antibiotics…More detailed studies of environmental reservoirs of resistance are crucial to our future ability to fight infection."

Al Naiemi, N., Duim, B., Savelkoul, P. H. M. et al. (2005). Widespread transfer of resistance genes between bacterial species in an intensive care unit: implications for hospital epidemiology. *Journal of Clinical Microbiology*. 43(9). pg. 4862-64. http://www.ncbi.nlm.nih.gov/pmc/articles/PMC1234139/

- "Recognition of plasmid transfer is crucial for control of outbreaks of multidrug-resistant nosocomial pathogens."

Altekruse, S. F., Stern, N. J., Fields, P. I. and Swerdlow, D. (1999). Campylobacter jejuni – An emerging foodborne pathogen. *Emerging Infectious Diseases*. 5(1). pg. 28-35. http://www.ncbi.nlm.nih.gov/pmc/articles/pmid/10081669/

- "*Campylobacter jejuni* is the most commonly reported bacterial cause of foodborne infection in the United States. Adding to the human and economic costs are chronic sequelae associated with *C. jejuni* infection – Guillian-Barre´syndrome and reactive arthritis."

- "Mishandling of raw poultry and consumption of undercooked poultry are the major risk factors for human campylobacteriosis. Efforts to prevent human illness are needed throughout each link in the food chain."
- The recent rapid spread of the mosquito before Zika virus has been noted by the CDC as sometimes associated with the presence of the Guillian-Barre´ syndrome (New York Times, 1/22/16).
- "In the United States, an estimated 2.1 to 2.4 million cases of human campylobacteriosis (illnesses ranging from loose stools to dysentery) occur each year."

Amabile-Cuevas, D. F. (2015) Antibiotics and antibiotic resistance in the environment. Routledge, NY.

American Academy of Microbiology. (2009). *Antibiotic resistance: An ecological perspective on an old problem.* http://academy.asm.org/images/stories/documents/antibioticresistance.pdf.

- "Humans are forced to coexist with the fact of antibiotic resistance. Public health officials, clinicians, and scientists must find effective ways to cope with antibiotic resistant bacteria harmful to humans and animals and to control the development of new types of resistance."
- "Exposure to antibiotics and other antimicrobial products, whether in the human body, in animals, or the environment, applies selective pressure that encourages resistance to emerge favoring both 'naturally resistant' strains and strains which have 'acquired resistance'."
- "Rapid diagnostic methods and surveillance are some of the most valuable tools in preventing the spread of resistance…A rigorous surveillance network to track the evolution and spread of resistance is also needed."

Aminov, R. I. (2009). The role of antibiotics and antibiotic resistance in nature. *Environmental Microbiology.* 11(12). pg. 2970-88. http://onlinelibrary.wiley.com/doi/10.1111/j.1462-2920.2009.01972.x/epdf

- "A broader overview of the role of antibiotics and antibiotic resistance in nature from the evolutionary and ecological prospective suggests that antibiotics have evolved as another way of intra- and inter-domain communication in various ecosystems."
- "The emergence and rapid dissemination of antibiotic-resistant pathogens, especially multi-drug-resistant bacteria, during recent decades, exposed our lack of knowledge about the evolutionary and ecological processes taking place in microbial ecosystems."

Andersson, D. I. and Hughes, D. (2011). Persistence of antibiotic resistance in bacterial populations. *FEMS Microbiology Reviews*. 35. pg. 901-11. http://femsre.oxfordjournals.org/cgi/pmidlookup?view=long&pmid=21707669

- "In this review, we discuss the multitude of mechanisms and processes that are involved in causing the persistence of chromosomal and plasmid-borne resistance determinants and how we might use them to our advantage to increase the likelihood of reversing the problem."
- "Very low antibiotic concentration can be enriching for resistant bacteria...antibiotic release into the environment could contribute to the selection for resistance."

Angier, Natalie. (October 28, 2014). Why viruses went viral: Ebola comes from a long line of cunning parasites, perhaps older than cells themselves. *The New York Times*. pg. D3. http://www.nytimes.com/2014/10/28/science/ebola-and-the-vast-viral-universe.html?_r=0

Apata, D. F. (2009). Antibiotic resistance in poultry. *Journal of Poultry Science*. 8(4). pg. 404-08. http://www.pjbs.org/ijps/fin1345.pdf

- "Sub therapeutic dosing in feed increase the rate of weight gain and improve the efficiency of converting feed to meat. The recommended levels of antibiotics in feed were 5-10 kg in the 1950's and have increased by ten to twenty folds since then."

Arias, C. A. and Murray, B. E. (2009). Antibiotic-resistant bugs in the 21st century – a clinical super-challenge. *The New England Journal of Medicine*. 360(5). pg. 439-43. http://www.nejm.org/doi/full/10.1056/NEJMp0804651

- "By 2003, more than 50% of *S. aureus* isolates recovered in U.S. hospitals were MRSA (methicillin-resistant *Staphylococcus aureus*)."
- "It is more difficult than ever to eradicate infections caused by antibiotic-resistant "superbugs," and the problem is exacerbated by a dry pipeline for new antimicrobials with bactericidal activity against gram-negative bacteria and enterococci."
- "A concerted effort on the part of academic researchers and their institutions, industry, and government is crucial if humans are to maintain the upper hand in this battle against bacteria – a fight with global consequences."

Armstrong, J. L., Shigeno, D. S., Calomiris, J. J. and Seidler, R. J. (1981). Antibiotic-resistant bacteria in drinking water. *Applied Environmental Microbiology*. 42. pg. 277-83. http://www.ncbi.nlm.nih.gov/pmc/articles/PMC244002/pdf/aem00189-0099.pdf

Ash, R., Mauck, B. and Morgan, M. (2002). Antibiotic resistance of gram-negative bacteria in rivers, United States. *Emerging Infectious Disease*. 8(7). pg. 713-6. http://www.ncbi.nlm.nih.gov/pmc/articles/PMC2730334/

- "Bacteria with intrinsic resistance to antibiotics are found in nature. Such organisms may acquire additional resistance genes from bacteria introduced into soil or water, and the resident bacteria may be the reservoir or source of widespread resistant organisms found in many environments."
- "We isolated antibiotic-resistant bacteria in freshwater samples from 16 U.S. rivers at 22 sites and measured the prevalence of organisms resistant to [beta]-lactam and non-[beta]-lactam antibiotics. Over 40% of the bacteria resistant to more than one antibiotic had at least one plasmid. Ampicillin resistance genes, as well as other resistance traits, were identified in 70% of the plasmids. The most common resistant organisms belonged to the following genera: Acinetobacter, Alciligenes, Citrobacter, Enterobacter, Pseudomonas, and Serratia."

Association for Professionals in Infection Control and Epidemiology (APIC). (2014). MRSA infection rates drop in veterans affairs long-term care facilities. *Infection Control Today*. http://www.infectioncontroltoday.com/news/2014/01/mrsa-infection-rates-drop-in-veterans-affairs-longterm-care-facilities.aspx

- "Four years after implementing a national initiative to reduce methicillin-resistant Staphylococcus aureus (MRSA) rates in Veterans Affairs (VA) long-term care facilities, MRSA infections have declined significantly, according to a study in the January issue of the American Journal of Infection Control, the official publication of the Association for Professionals in Infection Control and Epidemiology (APIC)."

Baam, B., Gandhi, N. and Freitas, Y. (1996). Antibiotic activity of marine microorganisms. *Helgoländer Wissenschaftliche Meeresuntersuchungen*. 13. pg. 181-5. http://link.springer.com/article/10.1007%2FBF01612663#page-1

Baquero, F., Martinez, J. and Canton, R. (2008) Antibiotics and antibiotic resistance in water environments. *Current Opinion in Biotechnology*. 19. pg. 260-5. http://www.ncbi.nlm.nih.gov/pubmed/18534838

Barraud, O., Casellas, M. Dagot, C. and Ploy, M-C. (2012). An antibiotic-resistant class 3 integron in an Enterobacter cloacae isolate from hospital effluent. *Clinical Microbiology and Infection*. 19. pg. E306-08. http://www.clinicalmicrobiologyandinfection.com/article/S1198-743X(14)61852-8/pdf

- "Class 3 integrons could thus be involved in the dissemination of antibiotic resistance in both clinical settings and the environment, and could participate in the exchange of antibiotic-resistance GCs between these two ecosystems."

Barrett, R., et al. (1998). Emerging and re-emerging infectious diseases: The third epidemiologic transition. *Annual Review of Anthropology.* 27. pg. 247-71. http://www.annualreviews.org/doi/abs/10.1146/annurev.anthro.27.1.247?journalCode=anthro

- "The first epidemiologic transition was associated with a rise in infectious diseases that accompanied the Neolithic Revolution."
- "The second epidemiologic transition involved the shift from infectious to chronic disease mortality associated with industrialization."
- "The recent resurgence of infectious disease mortality marks a third epidemiologic transition characterized by newly emerging, re-emerging, and antibiotic resistant pathogens in the context of an accelerated globalization of human disease ecologies."
- Contains a comprehensive bibliography pertaining to the sociohistory of human-disease relationships.

Bassetti, M., Repetto, E., Righi, E. et al (2008). Colistin and rifampicin in the treatment of multidrug-resistant Acinetobacter baumannii infections. *Journal of Antimicrobial Chemotherapy.* 61(2). pg. 417-20. http://jac.oxfordjournals.org/content/61/2/417.full

- "Colistin and rifampicin appears to be an effective and safe combination therapy for severe infections due to multidrug-resistant *A. baumannii.*"
- Written in 2007, this conclusion is no longer practical in most intensive care units (ICUs) in or after 2016.

Belluck, Pam. (May 10, 2016). Zika's secret assault: A race to unravel the secrets of the Zika virus. *The New York Times.* pg. D1. http://www.nytimes.com/2016/05/10/science/a-window-into-the-workings-of-zika.html?_r=0

- "A graduate student's offhand remark led to a remarkable finding about how the virus has caused lasting brain damage in so many babies."

Benotti, M. J., Trenholm, R. A., Vanderford, B. J., et al. (2009). Pharmaceuticals and endocrine disrupting compounds in U.S. drinking water. *Environmental Science & Technology.* 43(3). pg. 597-603. http://pubs.acs.org/doi/abs/10.1021/es801845a

- "The drinking water for more than 28 million people was screened for a diverse group of pharmaceuticals, potential endocrine disrupting compounds (EDCs), and other unregulated organic contaminants."
- "Source water, finished drinking water, and distribution system (tap) water from 19 U.S. water utilities was analyzed for 51 compounds between 2006 and 2007."
- "The 11 most frequently detected compounds were atenolol, atrazine, carbamazepine, estrone, gemfibrozil, meprobamate, naproxen, phenytoin, sulfamethoxazole, TCEP, and trimethoprim."
- Atrazine was detected in source waters far removed from agricultural application where wastewater was the only known source of organic contaminants."
- "Pharmaceuticals and endocrine disrupting compounds (EDCs) are subclasses of organic contaminants that have been detected in wastewater and surface waters throughout the world."
- "Their occurrence is most often a result of municipal wastewater discharge, as these compounds are not completely removed during treatment. Other sources of pharmaceuticals and EDCs in water include runoff from agricultural fields, concentrated animal feeding operations, landfill leachates, and urban runoff."

Bergstrom, C. T., Lo, M. and Lipstitch, M. (2004). Ecological theory suggests that antimicrobial cycling will not reduce antimicrobial resistance in hospitals. *PNAS*. 101(36). pg. 13285-90. http://www.pnas.org/content/101/36/13285.full

- "Alternative drug-use strategies such as mixing, in which each treated patient receives one of several drug classes used simultaneously in the hospitals, are predicted to be more effective."

Berry, D., Xi, C. and Raskin, L. (2006). Microbial ecology of drinking water distribution systems. *Current Opinions in Biotechnology*. 17. pg. 297-308. http://www.sciencedirect.com/science/article/pii/S0958166906000656

Bhullar, K., et al. (2012). Antibiotic resistance is prevalent in an isolated cave microbiome. *PLoS ONE*. 7(4). pg. 1-11. http://journals.plos.org/plosone/article?id=10.1371/journal.pone.0034953

- "A growing body of evidence implicates environmental organisms as reservoirs of these resistance genes…We report a screen of a sample of the culturable microbiome of Lechuguilla Cave, New Mexico. In a region of the cave that has been isolated for over 4 million years…some strains were resistant to 14 different commercially available antibiotics."

- "The prevalence of resistance, even in microbiomes isolated from human use of antibiotics…supports a growing understanding that antibiotic resistance is natural, ancient, and hard wired in the microbial pangenome."

Binder, S., Levitt, A. M., Sacks, J. J. and Hughes, J. M. (1999). Emerging infectious diseases: Public health issues for the 21st century. *Science*. 287. pg. 443-9. http://www.ncbi.nlm.nih.gov/pubmed/10334978

Bispo, P. J. M., Alfonso, E. C., Flynn, H. W. and Miller, D. (2013). Emerging 8-methoxyfluoroquinolone resistance among methicillin-susceptible staphylococcus epidermidis isolates recovered from patients with endophthalmitis. *Journal of Clinical Microbiology*. 51(9). pg. 2959-63. http://www.ncbi.nlm.nih.gov/pmc/articles/PMC3754617/

- "Fluoroquinolone resistance among staphylococci endophthalmitis isolates is a major and increasing concern in opthamology."
- "To prevent the growing resistance to the newer fluoroquinolones among staphylococci isolates from endophthalmitis cases, the extensive use of gatifloxacin and moxifloxacin pre-and postoperatively for the prevention of endophthalmitis should be reconsidered."

Blakeslee, S. (February 2, 2016). Post-cesarean bacteria transfer could change health for life, study shows. *The New York Times*.

- "The first germs to colonize a newborn delivered vaginally come almost exclusively from the mother. But the first to reach an infant born by cesarean section come mostly from the environment – particularly bacteria from inaccessible or less-scrubbed areas like lamps and walls, and from skin cells from everyone else in the delivery room."
- "Some epidemiological studies have suggested that C-section babies may have an elevated risk for developing immune and metabolic disorders, including Type 1 diabetes, allergies, asthma and obesity."
- "Scientists have theorized that these children may be missing key bacteria known to play a large role in shaping the immune system from the moment of birth onward."

Blaser, Martin. (2015). *Missing microbes: How the overuse of antibiotics is fueling our modern plague*. Picadore, Henry Holton Co., NY.

- "In 1850, one in four American babies died before his or her first birthday. Lethal epidemics swept through crowded cities, as people were packed into dark, dirty rooms with fetid air and no running water. Familiar scourges included cholera, pneumonia, scarlet fever, diphtheria, whooping cough, tuberculosis and smallpox. Today, only six in every thousand infants in the United States are expected to die before age one."

- "We are suffering from a mysterious array of what I call 'modern plagues': obesity, childhood diabetes, asthma, hay fever, food allergies, esophageal reflux and cancer, celiac, Crohn's Disease, ulcer colitis, autism, and eczema."
- "These disorders suggest that our children are experiencing levels of immune dysfunction never seen before, as well as conditions such as autism…"
- "Each of us hosts a…diverse ecology of microbes that has evolved with our species over millennia…the microbes that constitute your microbiome are generally acquired early in life; surprisingly, by the age of three."
- "Loss of diversity within our microbiome…changes development itself, affecting our metabolism, immunity, and cognition."
- "We are losing our ancient microbes…the loss of microbial diversity on and within our bodies is exacting a terrible price. I predict it will be worse in the future."
- "An even worse scenario is headed our way if we don't change our behavior. It is one so bleak…that I call it 'antibiotic winter.'"
- "Ancient microbes, missing from us, might be used to protect our children from the modern diseases now plaguing…us as a result of our exposure to antibiotics and other aspects of medical care and, indeed, of modern life…as with fecal transfers, the idea is to somehow restore the missing microbes."

Blinder, Alan. (September 2, 2016). Aimed at Zika mosquitoes, spray kills millions of bees. *The New York Times*. pg. A11. http://www.nytimes.com/2016/09/02/us/south-carolina-pesticide-kills-bees.html?_r=0

Bonomo, R. A. (2000). Multiple antibiotic-resistant bacteria in long-term-care facilities: an emerging problem in the practice of infectious diseases. *Clinical Infectious Diseases*. 31(6). pg. 1414-22. http://cid.oxfordjournals.org/content/31/6/1414.long

- "Because of the increased infection rate antibiotics account for nearly 40% of all medications prescribed in LTCFs. Predictably, antibiotic-resistant pathogens are frequently being recovered in these settings."

Boyd, G., Reemtsma, H., Grimm, D. A., et al. (2003). Pharmaceuticals and personal care products (PPCPs) in surface and treated waters of Louisiana, USA and Ontario, Canada. *Science of the Total Environment*. 311(1). pg. 145-9. http://www.sciencedirect.com/science/article/pii/S0048969703001384

Bradley, P., Barber, L., Duris, J., et al. (2014). Riverbank filtration potential of pharmaceuticals in a wastewater-impacted stream. *Environmental Pollution*. 193. pg.

173-80. http://ac.els-cdn.com/S0269749114002607/1-s2.0-S0269749114002607-main.pdf?_tid=5a016a38-aedb-11e4-a360-00000aab0f6b&acdnat=1423321965_583f2d8d2cb12191a71d019a0387e135

- Research conducted in October and December 2012.
- "The results demonstrate the importance of effluent discharge as a driver of local hydrologic conditions in an effluent-impacted stream and thus as a fundamental control on surface-water to groundwater transport of effluent-derived pharmaceutical contaminants."
- "Wastewater reuse is necessary to meet current and future downstream-flow requirements and other water-supply demands, but inevitably increases the risks of aquatic ecosystem impairment and contamination of surface-water and groundwater drinking-water supplies."
- "Wastewater contaminants raise fundamental concerns due to the chemical and biological complexity of wastewater mixtures, the potential for introduction into water resources, and the wide range of ecological and human health impacts."
- "Wastewater pharmaceuticals are especially challenging due to their: relative solubility and high mobility in aqueous environments compared with many other wastewater contaminants; designed high bioactivities and long shelf-lives (biorecalcitrance); and wide range of potential ecological endpoints including toxicity, endocrine disruption, immune-modulation, antibiotic resistance selection, as well as cytotoxicity and mutagenesis."

Bryce, A., Hay, A. D., Lane, I. F. et al. (2016). Global prevalence of antibiotic resistance in paediatric urinary tract infections caused by *Escherichia coli* and association with routine use of antibiotics in primary care: Systematic review and meta-analysis. *BMJ*. 352. http://www.bmj.com/content/352/bmj.i939

California Healthcare Institute (2011). *Promoting antibiotic discovery and development: A California healthcare institute initiative.* http://www.chi.org/uploadedFiles/Industry_at_a_glance/CHI%20Antibiotic%20White%20Paper_FINAL.pdf

- "The U.S. Food and Drug Administration (FDA) has the power and the ability to solve this problem. This is because the most important barrier to industry investment is the FDA regulatory process."
- "The RandD time for taking a new molecule from identification to clinical use is typically about eight years…The pharmaceutical industry views the current state of FDA regulation of antibiotics as uncertain and unduly risky."

- "The rapid emergence on a global basis of bacteria resistant to all known antibiotics has created a looming public health crisis that is affecting all hospitals and communities in the U.S. Regulatory and market forces have led to an exodus of major pharmaceutical companies from the field."
- CHI is probably a California biomedical community sponsored institute.

Canton, R., Friedrich, A., Poirel, L. et al. (2013). Carbapenemase-producing Enterobacteriaceae in Europe: A survey among national experts from 39 countries, February 2013. *European Communicable Disease Bulletin.* 7. www.eurosurveillance.org.

- "Thirty three of the NEs indicated that *Klebsiella pneumoniae* was the most frequent *Enterobacteriaceae* species to produce carbapenemases in their country. Overall, *K. pneumoniae* carbapenemase-producing *Enterobacteriaceae* (KPC) have attained the widest distribution…The true extent of CPE occurrence in Europe is still underestimated."

Capita, R., Riesco-Pelaez, F., Alonso-Hernando, A. and Alonso-Calleja, C. (2013). Exposure to sub-lethal concentrations of food-grade biocides influences the ability to form biofilm, the resistance to antimicrobials and the ultrastructure of *Escherichia coli* ATCC 12806. *Applied Environmental Microbiology.* 80(4). pg. 1268-80. http://www.asm.org/images/Communications/tips/2014/0114biocide.pdf

- "Escherichia coli ATCC 12806 was exposed to increasing sub-inhibitory concentrations of three biocides widely used in food industry facilities: trisodium phosphate (TSP), sodium nitrite (SNI) and sodium hypochlorite (SHY). The cultures exhibited an acquired tolerance to biocides (especially to SNI and SHY) after exposure to such compounds…TSP reduced the ability of E. coli to produce biofilm."
- "Cultures exposed to biocides displayed a stable reduced susceptibility to a range of antibiotics (mainly aminoglycosides, cephalosporins and quinolones), as compared with cultures not exposed. SNI caused the greatest 38 increase in resistances antibiotics; 48.3% of total…The findings of the present study suggest that the use of biocides at sub-inhibitory concentrations could represent a public health risk."

Carlet, J., Jarlier, V., Harbath, S., et al. (2012). Ready for a world without antibiotics? The Pensieres antibiotic resistance call to action. *Antimicrobial Resistance and Infection Control.* 1(11). pg. 1-13. http://www.ncbi.nlm.nih.gov/pmc/articles/PMC3436635/

- "Resistance to antibiotics has increased dramatically over the past few years and has now reached a level that places future patients in real danger."
- "To meet this challenge, 70 internationally recognized experts met for a two-day meeting in June 2011 in Annecy (France) and endorsed a global call to action ('The Pensieres Antibiotic Resistance Call to Action'). Bundles of measures that must be implemented simultaneously and worldwide are presented in this document. In particular, antibiotics, which represent a treasure for humanity, must be protected and considered as a special class of drugs."

Caruffo, M. and Navarette, P. (2015). Antibiotics in aquaculture: Impacts and alternatives. *The APUA Newsletter.* 3(2). pg. 4-7, 13. http://www.tufts.edu/med/apua/news/newsletter_71_523284685.pdf

- "Table 1: Alternatives to antibiotics in aquaculture; major advantages and limitations" cites the following "Antibiotic alternative: Antimicrobial peptides, Phage therapy, Short-cahin fatty acids, Bacteriocins, Probiotics, Prebiotics, [and] Essential oils (EOs)."

Casewell, M., et al. (2003). The European ban on growth-promoting antibiotics and emerging consequences for human and animal health. *Journal of Antimicrobial Chemotherapy.* 52. pg. 159-61. http://jac.oxfordjournals.org/content/52/2/159.full

- "A directly attributable effect of these infections is the increase in usage of therapeutic antibiotics in food animals, including that of tetracycline, aminoglycosides, trimethoprim/sulphonamide, macrolides and lincosamides, all of which are of direct importance in human medicine. The theoretical and political benefit of the widespread ban of growth promoters needs to be more carefully weighed against the increasingly apparent adverse consequences."

Centers for Disease Control and Prevention. (2004). *National antimicrobial resistance monitoring system for enteric bacteria (NARMS): 2002 human isolates final report.* U.S. Department of Health and Human Services, CDC, Atlanta, GA. http://www.cdc.gov/narms/annual/2002/2002ANNUALREPORTFINAL.pdf

Centers for Disease Control and Prevention. (2011). *A CDC framework for preventing infectious diseases.* CDC. http://www.cdc.gov/oid/docs/ID-Framework.pdf

- "Infectious diseases are a leading cause of illness and death throughout the world. The enormous diversity of microbes combined with their ability to evolve and adapt to changing populations, environments, practices, and technologies creates ongoing threats to health and continually challenges our efforts to prevent and control infectious diseases. A CDC Framework for Preventing Infectious

Diseases: Sustaining the Essentials and Innovating for the Future —CDC's ID Framework —was developed to provide a roadmap for improving our ability to prevent known infectious diseases and to recognize and control rare, highly dangerous, and newly emerging threats, through a strengthened, adaptable, and multi - purpose U.S. public health system. Although its primary purpose is to guide CDC's infectious disease activities, the document is also designed to guide collective public health action at a time of resource constraints and difficult decisions, while advancing opportunities to improve the nation's health through new ideas, partnerships, technical innovations, validated tools, and evidence - based policies. The ID Framework outlines three critical elements in these efforts: strong public health fundamentals, including infectious disease surveillance, laboratory detection, and epidemiologic investigation; high - impact interventions; and sound health policies . The document also describes priority activities for achieving these essential components of public health, highlighting opportunities afforded through scientific and technological innovations, new partnerships, and the changing U.S. public health and healthcare systems."

Centers for Disease Control and Prevention. (2012). *Cephalosporin-resistant Neisseria gonorrhoeae public health response plan*. CDC. www.cdc.gov/std/gonorrhea/default.htm

Centers for Disease Control and Prevention. (2013). *Antibiotic resistance threats in the United States, 2013*. CDC. http://www.cdc.gov/drugresistance/threat-report-2013/index.html

- "This report, Antibiotic resistance threats in the United States, 2013 gives a first-ever snapshot of the burden and threats posed by the antibiotic-resistant germs having the most impact on human health. Each year in the United States, at least 2 million people become infected with bacteria that are resistant to antibiotics and at least 23,000 people die each year as a direct result of these infections. Many more people die from other conditions that were complicated by an antibiotic-resistant infection. Antibiotic-resistant infections can happen anywhere. Data show that most happen in the general community; however, most deaths related to antibiotic resistance happen in healthcare settings such as hospitals and nursing homes."

Centers for Disease Control and Prevention. (2014). *Trends in tuberculosis, 2014*. CDC. http://www.cdc.gov/tb/publications/factsheets/statistics/tbtrends-2014.pdf

How many cases of tuberculosis (TB) were reported in the United States in 2014?

A total of 9,421 TB cases (a rate of 2.96 cases per 100,000 persons) were reported in the United States in 2014. Both the number of TB cases reported and the case rate decreased; this represents a 1.5% and 2.2% decline, respectively, compared to 2013.* This is the smallest decline in more than a decade.

*Ratio calculation is based on unrounded data values.

Is the rate of TB declining in the United States?

Yes. Since the 1992 peak of TB resurgence in the United States, the number of TB cases reported each year has decreased.

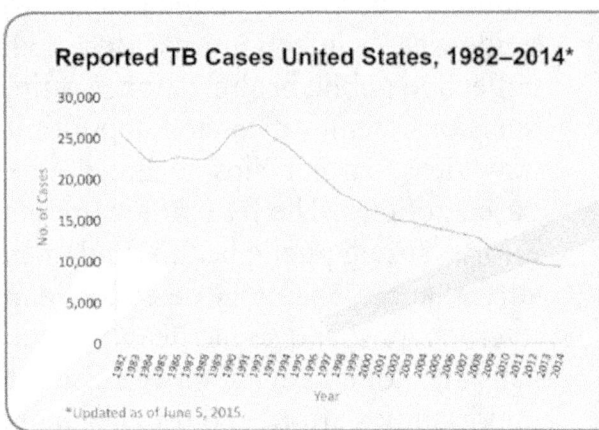

Reported TB Cases United States, 1982–2014*

No. of Cases

30,000
25,000
20,000
15,000
10,000
5,000
0

Year

*Updated as of June 5, 2015.

How do the TB rates compare between U.S.-born persons and foreign-born persons living in the United States?

In 2014, a total of 66% of reported TB cases in the United States occurred among foreign-born persons. The TB case rate among foreign-born persons (15.4 cases per 100,000 persons) in 2014 was approximately 13 times higher than among U.S.-born persons (1.2 cases per 100,000 persons).

How many people died from TB in the United States?

There were 555 deaths from TB in 2013, the most recent year for which these data are available. This is an 8% increase from the 510 TB deaths in 2012. Overall, the number of TB deaths reported annually has decreased by 67% since 1992.

What are the rates of TB for different racial and ethnic populations[†]?

- American Indians or Alaska Natives: 5.0 TB cases per 100,000 persons
- Asians: 17.8 TB cases per 100,000 persons
- Blacks or African Americans: 5.1 TB cases per 100,000 persons
- Native Hawaiians and other Pacific Islanders: 16.9 TB cases per 100,000 persons
- Hispanics or Latinos: 5.0 TB cases per 100,000 persons
- Whites: 0.6 TB cases per 100,000 persons

† For this report, persons identified as white, black, Asian, American Indian/Alaska Native, native Hawaiian or other Pacific Islander, or of multiple races are all non-Hispanic. Persons identified as Hispanic may be of any race.

TB Case Rates,* United States, 2014

D.C.

☐ ≤ 3.0 (2014 national average)
■ >3.0

*Cases per 100,000.

Is multidrug-resistant tuberculosis (MDR TB)* on the rise?

Overall, the percentage of MDR TB cases decreased slightly from 1.4% (96 cases) in 2013 to 1.3% (91 cases) in 2014.**

Of the total number of reported MDR TB cases, the proportion occurring among foreign-born persons increased from 31% (149 of 484) in 1993 to 88% (80 of 91) in 2014.

* MDR TB is defined as TB disease that is resistant to at least isoniazid and rifampin.

** Among culture-positive TB cases in the United States with initial drug-susceptibility testing results.

Where can I find TB data for my state?

The most recent surveillance report, *Reported Tuberculosis in the United States, 2014*, includes data from 60 reporting areas (the 50 states, the District of Columbia, New York City, Puerto Rico, and seven other U.S. jurisdictions in the Pacific and Caribbean). The report can be found online at http://www.cdc.gov/tb/statistics/default.htm. If you need additional state-specific data not available in this report, you can contact your state TB control office: http://www.cdc.gov/tb/links/tboffices.htm.

- **National Center for HIV/AIDS, Viral Hepatitis, STD, and TB Prevention (NCHHSTP) Atlas (2008-2013).** NCHHSTP Atlas is an interactive tool that allows users to observe trends and patterns by creating detailed reports, maps, and other graphics showing geographic patterns and time trends. Available at http://www.cdc.gov/nchhstp/atlas/.
- **Online Tuberculosis Information System (OTIS) (2009-2013).** OTIS is an interactive data system containing information on TB cases reported to CDC. Users can select criteria to produce specific reports. Data are available by year, state, and demographic factors. Available at http://wonder.cdc.gov/tb.html.

References

CDC. *Reported Tuberculosis in the United States, 2014*. Atlanta, GA: U.S. Department of Health and Human Services, CDC, October 2015. http://www.cdc.gov/tb/statistics/reports/2014

Additional Information

CDC. Questions and Answers About TB
http://www.cdc.gov/tb/publications/faqs/default.htm

CDC. The Difference Between Latent TB Infection and TB Disease
http://www.cdc.gov/tb/publications/factsheets/general/LTBIandActiveTB.htm

CDC. Multidrug-Resistant Tuberculosis
http://www.cdc.gov/tb/publications/factsheets/drtb/mdrtb.htm

State TB Control Offices
http://www.cdc.gov/tb/links/tboffices.htm

Centers for Disease Control and Prevention. (2015a). *Antibiotic-resistant gonorrhea.* CDC. http://www.cdc.gov/std/gonorrhea/arg/

- "The emergence of multidrug- and cephalosporin-resistant gonorrhea in the United States would make gonorrhea much more difficult to treat. Gonorrhea has progressively developed resistance to the antibiotic drugs prescribed to treat it.

Following the spread of gonococcal fluoroquinolone resistance, the cephalosporin antibiotics have been the foundation of recommended treatment for gonorrhea. The emergence of cephalosporin-resistant gonorrhea would significantly complicate the ability of providers to treat gonorrhea successfully, since we have few antibiotic options left that are simple, well-studied, well-tolerated and highly effective. It is critical to continuously monitor antibiotic resistance in *Neisseria gonorrhoeae* and encourage research and development of new treatment regimens.

Centers for Disease Control and Prevention. (2015b). *Antibiotic-resistant gonorrhea basic information*. CDC. http://www.cdc.gov/std/gonorrhea/arg/basic.htm

- Antibiotic resistance (AR) is the ability of bacteria to resist the effects of the drugs used to treat them. This means the germs are not killed and they will continue to reproduce. Neisseria (N.) gonorrhoeae, the bacteria that cause the STD gonorrhea, has developed resistance to nearly all of the antibiotics used for gonorrhea treatment: sulfonilamides, penicillin, tetracycline, and fluoroquinolones, such as ciprofloxacin. We are currently down to one last effective class of antibiotics, cephalosporins, to treat this common infection. This is an urgent public health threat because gonorrhea control in the United States largely relies on effective antibiotic therapy.

  Given the bacteria's ability to adapt and survive antibiotics, it is critical to continuously monitor for antibiotic resistance and encourage research and development of new treatment regimens for gonorrhea.

Surveillance

Surveillance for antimicrobial resistance in N. gonorrhoeae in the United States is conducted through the Gonococcal Isolate Surveillance Project (GISP). Each year, 25–30 sites and 4–5 regional laboratories across the United States participate in GISP and collect thousands of N. gonorrhoeae samples from men with urethral gonorrhea at STD clinics. Isolates from these samples are then used by researchers to determine the bacteria's susceptibility to a given set of antibiotics. Since 1989, data from this project have directly contributed to updating CDC's STD Treatment Guidelines for gonorrhea.

Clinicians are asked to report any N. gonorrhoeae specimen with decreased cephalosporin susceptibility and any gonorrhea cephalosporin treatment failure to CDC through their state or local public health authority. Bacteria have decreased susceptibility to a given antibiotic when laboratory results indicate that higher-than-expected antibiotic concentrations are needed to stop their growth.

In the United States, reports of apparent failures of infections to respond to treatment with CDC-recommended therapies should be reported to Robert D. Kirkcaldy, MD, MPH (rkirkcaldy@cdc.gov; 404-639-8659), Surveillance & Data Management Branch, Division of STD Prevention, Centers for Disease Control and Prevention, 1600 Clifton Rd. NE, Mailstop E02, Atlanta, GA 30333.

CDC also recommends that isolates from certain infections be submitted to the Neisseria Reference Laboratory at CDC for confirmation: John Papp, Ph.D. JPapp@cdc.gov; 404-639-3785, Neisseria Reference Laboratory, Centers for Disease Control and Prevention, 1600 Clifton Rd. NE, Mailstop A12, Atlanta, GA 30333. These infections comprise those that do not respond to CDC-recommended therapy. See pg. 6, Recommended Testing and Confirmatory Testing for a complete list.

Trends and Treatment

In 1993, ciprofloxacin, a fluoroquinolone, and cephalosporins ceftriaxone and cefixime were the recommended treatments for gonorrhea. However, in the late 1990s and early 2000s, ciprofloxacin resistance was detected in Hawaii and the West Coast, and by 2004 ciprofloxacin resistance was detected among men who have sex with men (MSM) with gonorrhea. By 2006, 13.8% of isolates exhibited resistance to ciprofloxacin, and ciprofloxacin resistance was present in all regions of the country, and in the heterosexual population. On April 13, 2007, CDC stopped recommending fluoroquinolones as empiric treatment for gonococcal infections for all people in the United States. The cephalosporins, either cefixime or ceftriaxone, were the only remaining recommended treatments.

Similar to trends observed elsewhere in the world, CDC has observed recent worrisome trends of decreasing cephalosporin susceptibility, especially to the oral cephalosporin cefixime. To preserve cephalosporins for as long as possible, CDC has since then made the following changes to its STD Treatment Guidelines:

In 2010, CDC changed its treatment recommendations to recommend dual therapy for the treatment of gonorrhea and increased the recommended dose of ceftriaxone to 250 mg.

Following continued declines in cefixime susceptibility, CDC updated its recommendations in 2012 to recommend ceftriaxone plus either azithromycin or doxycycline as the only first-line treatment.

CDC's 2015 STD Treatment Guidelines now recommend only one regimen of dual therapy for the treatment of gonorrhea—the injectable cephalosporin ceftriaxone, plus oral azithromycin. Dual therapy is recommended to address the potential emergence of gonococcal cephalosporin resistance.

In 2012 and 2013, there were dramatic decreases in resistance to cefixime. However, resistance levels increased in 2014. CDC has not received any reports of verified clinical treatment failures to any cephalosporin in the United States.

Challenges

A major challenge to monitoring emerging antimicrobial resistance of N. gonorrhoeae is the substantial decline in the use of gonorrhea culture by many clinicians, as well as the reduced capability of many laboratories to perform gonorrhea culture techniques required for antibiotic susceptibility testing. Culture testing is when the bacteria is first grown on a nutrient plate and is then exposed to known amounts of an antibiotic to determine the bacteria's susceptibility to the antibiotic. The decline in culture testing results from an increased use of newer nonculture-based laboratory technology, such as a diagnostic test called the Nucleic Acid Amplification Test (NAAT). Currently, there is no well-studied reliable technology that allows for antibiotic susceptibility testing from nonculture specimens. Increased laboratory culture capacity is needed.

Laboratory Issues

CDC recommends that all state and local health department labs maintain or develop the capacity to perform gonorrhea culture, or form partnerships with experienced laboratories that can perform this type of testing.

Centers for Disease Control and Prevention. (2015c). *Nearly half a million Americans suffered from Clostridium difficile infections in a single year*. CDC. http://www.cdc.gov/media/releases/2015/p0225-clostridium-difficile.html

- *"Clostridium difficile (C. difficile)* caused almost half a million infections among patients in the United States in a single year, according to a study released today by the Centers for Disease Control and Prevention (CDC)… *C. difficile* causes an inflammation of the color and deadly diarrhea."

- "Approximately 29,000 patients died within 30 days of the initial diagnosis of *C. difficile*…More than 80 percent of the deaths associated with *C. difficile* occurred among Americans aged 65 years or older."
- "1 out of every 5 patients with a healthcare-associated *C. difficile* infection experienced a recurrence of the infection and 1 out of every 9 patients aged 65 or older with a healthcare-associated *C. difficile* infection died within 30 days of diagnosis."

Centers for Disease Control and Prevention. (2016a). *Antibiotic resistance solutions initiative*. CDC. http://www.cdc.gov/budget/documents/fy2016/antibiotic-resistance-factsheet.pdf

Centers for Disease Control and Prevention. (2016b). *Draft interim CDC Zika response plan (CONUS and Hawaii): Initial response to Zika Virus*. CDC, Atlanta, Georgia. https://www.cdc.gov/zika/pdfs/zika-draft-interim-conus-plan.pdf

- See Appendix 6: Zika: CDC Draft Interim Response Plan for a copy of the table of contents and purpose.

Ceylan, O., Okemen, G. and Ugur, A. (2008). Isolation of soil streptomyces as source antibiotics active against antibiotic-resistant bacteria. *Journal of Biosciences*. pg. 73-82. www.ejobios.com/content/2/9/73-82. http://citeseerx.ist.psu.edu/viewdoc/download?doi=10.1.1.549.3449&rep=rep1&type=pdf

- "In this work, we have shown that a total of 15 different *Streptomycetes* isolates associated with soil have the ability to produce antimicrobial compounds against microorganisms, especially multiple antibiotic resistant Gram positive and Gram negative bacteria. Further investigations are needed in order to further determine the active metabolites of these isolates."

Chen, M., Yu, Q. and Sun, H. (2013). Novel strategies for the prevention and treatment of biofilm related infections. *International Journal of Molecular Sciences*. 14. pg. 18488-501.

- "Biofilm formation by human bacterial pathogens on implanted medical devices causes major morbidity and mortality among patients, and leads to billions of dollars in healthcare cost. Biofilm is a complex bacterial community that is highly resistant to antibiotics and human immunity."
- "As a result, novel therapeutic solutions other than the conventional antibiotic therapies are in urgent need…Discovery of alternative approaches to prevent or

treat biofilms...[includes] the molecular mechanism of biofilm formation [and] modifying the biomaterials used in medical devices."

- "These novel anti-biofilm technologies could eventually lead to anti-biofilm therapies that are superior to the current antibiotic treatment."

Choffnes, Eileen R., Relman, David A., Olsen, LeighAnne, Hutton, Rebekah and Mack, Alison, eds. (2012). *Improving food safety through a one health approach: Workshop summary.* The National Academies Press, Washington, DC. http://www.ncbi.nlm.nih.gov/books/NBK100665/pdf/Bookshelf_NBK100665.pdf

Cole, M., et al. (2014). Emerging cephalosporin and multidrug-resistant gonorrhea in Europe. *Surveillance and Outbreak Reports.* 19(45). pg. 1-5. http://www.eurosurveillance.org/images/dynamic/EE/V19N45/art20955.pdf

- "Since 2009 the European gonococcal antimicrobial surveillance programme (Euro-GASP) has been running as a sentinel surveillance system across Member States of the European Union (EU) and European Economic Area (EEA) to monitor antimicrobial susceptibility in *N. gonorrhoeae*."
- "During 2011 *N. gonorrhoeae* isolates were collected from 21 participating countries...the rate of ciprofloxacin and azithromycin resistance was 48.7% and 5.3%, respectively."

Collignon, P., Athukorala, P-C, Senanayake, S. and Khan, F. (2015). Antimicrobial resistance: The major contribution of poor governance and corruption to this growing problem. *PLOS One.* pg. 1-13. http://journals.plos.org/plosone/article?id=10.1371/journal.pone.0116746

- "Increasing resistance involves nearly all bacteria that infect people, including very common ones such as *Escherichia coli* and *Staphylococcus aureus*."
- "Poor infection control, poor water sanitation and poor hygiene all facilitate the spread of resistant bacteria from person to person. The majority of antibiotic usage worldwide is in food animals. This usage leads to the development of resistant bacteria, which spread to people via the food chain and/or water."
- "Only 28% of the total variation in antibiotic resistance among countries is attributable to variation in antibiotic usage...However when the control of corruption indicator is included as an additional variable, 63% of the total variation in antibiotic resistance is now explained by the regression...indicating that corruption is the main socioeconomic factor that explains antibiotic resistance."

Table 1. *Critically important* antimicrobials that are used in human medicine.

Antimicrobial class	Antimicrobial(s)	Criterion 1[a]	Criterion 2[b]	Comment(s)
Aminoglycosides	Amikacin and arbekacin; gentamicin, netilmicin, and tobramycin; and streptomycin	Yes	Yes	Limited therapy as part of treatment of enterococcal endocarditis and MDR tuberculosis Potential transmission of *Enterococcus* species, Enterobacteriaceae (including *Escherichia coli*), and *Mycobacterium* species from nonhuman sources.
Ansamycins	Rifabutin, rifampin, and rifaximin	Yes	Yes	Limited therapy as part of therapy of mycobacterial diseases including tuberculosis and single drug therapy may select for resistance Potential transmission of *Mycobacterium* species from nonhuman sources
Carbapenems and other penems	Ertapenem, faropenem, imipenem, and meropenem	Yes	Yes	Limited therapy as part of treatment of disease due to MDR gram-negative bacteria Potential transmission of Enterobacteriaceae, including *E. coli* and *Salmonella* sprecies, from nonhuman sources
Cephalosporins, third and fourth generation	Cefixime, cefotaxime, cefpodoxime, ceftazidime, ceftizoxime, cefoperazone, cefoperazone-sulbactam, and ceftriaxone; cefepime, cefpirome, and cefoselis	Yes	Yes	Limited therapy for acute bacterial meningitis and disease due to *Salmonella* in children Fourth-generation cephalosporins provide limited therapy for empirical treatment of neutropenic patients with persistent fever Potential transmission of Enterobacteriaceae, including *E. coli* and *Salmonella* species, from nonhuman sources
Glycopeptides	Teicoplanin and vancomycin	Yes	Yes	Limited therapy for infection due to MDR *Staphylococcus aureus* and *Enterococcus* species Potential transmission of *Enterococcus* species and MDR *S. aureus* from nonhuman sources
Lipopeptides	Daptomycin	Yes	Yes	Limited therapy for infection due to MDR *S. aureus* Potential transmission of *Enterococcus* species and MDR *S. aureus* from nonhuman sources
Macrolides, including 14-, 15-, and 16-membered compounds, and ketolides	Azithromycin, clarithromycin, erythromycin, midecamycin, roxithromycin, spiramycin, and telithromycin	Yes	Yes	Limited therapy for infection due to *Legionella*, *Campylobacter*, and MDR *Salmonella* species Potential transmission of *Campylobacter* species from nonhuman sources
Oxazolidinones	Linezolid	Yes	Yes	Limited therapy for infection due to MDR *S. aureus* and *Enterococcus* species Potential transmission of *Enterococcus* species and MDR *S. aureus* from nonhuman sources
Penicillins, including natural penicillins, aminopenicillins, and antipseudomonals	Penicillin G, penicillin V, ampicillin, ampicillin-sulbactam, amoxicillin, amoxicillin-clavulanate, piperacillin, piperacillin-tazobactam, azlocillin, carbenicillin, mezlocillin, ticarcillin, and ticarcillin-clavulanate	Yes	Yes	Limited therapy for syphilis (natural penicillins), *Listeria* and *Enterococcus* species (aminopenicillins), and MDR *Pseudomonas* species (antipseudomonals) Potential transmission of *Enterococcus* species, Enterobacteriaceae (including *E. coli*, and *Pseudomonas aeruginosa* from nonhuman sources
Quinolones	Cinoxacin, nalidixic acid, and pipemidic acid; ciprofloxacin, enoxacin, gatifloxacin, gemifloxacin, levofloxacin, lomefloxacin, moxifloxacin, norfloxacin, ofloxacin, and sparfloxacin	Yes	Yes	Limited therapy for *Campylobacter* species, invasive disease due to *Salmonella* species, and MDR *Shigella* species infection Potential transmission of *Campylobacter* species and Enterobacteriaceae, including *E. coli* and *Salmonella* species, from nonhuman sources
Streptogramins	quinupristin-dalfopristin and pristinamycin	Yes	Yes	Limited therapy for MDR *Enterococcus faecium* and *S. aureus* infection Potential transmission of *Enterococcus* species and MDR *S. aureus* from nonhuman sources
Tetracyclines and glycylcyclines	Tigecycline	Yes	Yes	Limited therapy for infection due to MDR *S. aureus*

33

Table 2. *Highly important* antimicrobials that are used in human medicine.

Antimicrobial class	Antimicrobial(s)	Criterion 1[a]	Criterion 2[b]	Comment(s)
Amidinopenicillins	Mecillinam	No[c]	Yes	Potential transmission of Enterobacteriaceae, including *Escherichia coli*, from nonhuman sources MDR *Shigella* species infections may be a regional problem.
Aminoglycosides, other	Kanamycin, neomycin, and spectinomycin	No	Yes	Potential transmission of gram-negative bacteria that are cross-resistant to streptomycin from nonhuman sources
Amphenicols	Chloramphenicol and thiamphenicol	No[c]	Yes	May be 1 of limited therapies for acute bacterial meningitis, typhoid fever, and respiratory infections in certain geographic areas
Cephalosporins, first and second generation	Cefazolin, cephalexin, cephalothin, and cephradine	No	Yes	Potential transmission of Enterobacteriaceae, including *E. coli*, from nonhuman sources
Cephalosporins, second generation	Cefaclor, cefamandole, cefuroxime, and loracarbef	No	Yes	Potential transmission of Enterobacteriaceae, including *E. coli*, from non-human sources
Cephamycins	Cefotetan and cefoxitin	No	Yes	Potential transmission of Enterobacteriaceae, including *E. coli*, from nonhuman sources
Clofazimine	Clofazimine	Yes	No	Limited therapy for leprosy
Monobactams	Aztreonam	No	Yes	Potential transmission of Enterobacteriaceae, including *E. coli*, from nonhuman sources
Penicillins, antistaphylococcals	Cloxacillin, dicloxacillin, flucloxacillin, oxacillin, and nafcillin	No	Yes	*Staphylococcus aureus*, including methicillin-resistant *S. aureus*, has been transferred to humans from animals
Polymyxins	Colistin and polymyxin B	Yes	No	Polymyxins may be the only available therapy for some infections due to gram-negative bacteria (e.g., infection due to *Acinetobacter* species and *Pseudomonas aeruginosa*)
Sulfonamides, dihydrofolate reductase inhibitors, and combinations	Para-aminobenzoic acid, pyrimethamine, sulfadiazine, sulfamethoxazole, sulfapyridine, sulfisoxazole, and trimethoprim	No[c]	Yes	Potential transmission of Enterobacteriaceae, including *E. coli*, from nonhuman sources May be 1 of limited therapies for acute bacterial meningitis and other infections in certain geographic areas
Sulfones	Dapsone	Yes	No	Limited therapy for leprosy
Tetracyclines	Chlortetracycline, doxycycline, minocycline, oxytetracycline, and tetracycline	Yes	No	Limited therapy for infection due to *Chlamydia* species and *Rickettsia* species

NOTE. From the World Health Organization meeting in Copenhagen, Denmark [18]. One of the 2 following criteria were met for classification as a *highly important* antimicrobial: (1) the agent or class is the sole therapy or one of few alternatives to treat serious human disease; and (2) the antimicrobial agent or class is used to treat diseases caused by organisms that may be transmitted via nonhuman sources or diseases causes by organisms that may acquire resistance genes from nonhuman sources. MDR, multidrug-resistant.

[a] Criterion 1: the agent or class is the sole therapy or one of few alternatives to treat serious human disease.

[b] Criterion 2: the antimicrobial agent or class is used to treat diseases caused by organisms that may be transmitted via nonhuman sources or diseases causes by organisms that may acquire resistance genes from nonhuman sources.

[c] The importance of the class or antimicrobial may change on the basis of regional differences.

Collignon, P., Power, J., Chiller, T. M., et al. (2009). World Health Organization ranking of antimicrobials according to their importance in human medicine: a critical step for developing risk management strategies for the use of antimicrobials in food production animals. *Clinical Infectious Disease.* 49(1). pg. 132-41. http://cid.oxfordjournals.org/content/49/1/132.long

- "Improved management of the use of antimicrobials in food animals, particularly reducing the usage of those that are 'critically important' for human medicine, is an important step toward preserving the benefits of antimicrobials for people."
- "Poverty; suboptimal control of the sale, quality, and use of antimicrobials; and poor sewage and water systems are factors that contribute to the emergence and spread of antimicrobial resistance."
- "The US Food and Drug Administration (FDA) has been particularly concerned about the extra-label use of cephalosporins (e.g., ceftiofur) in food animals, especially poultry…[which] has contributed to emerging cephalosporin-resistant zoonotic foodborne bacteria."
- Once the gene is established in a successful virulent clone, the clone and the carried gene can spread in individual countries and worldwide, such as in the case of multidrug-resistant *S. aureus* and pneumococci."

Conlon, B., Nakayasu, E., Fleck, L., et al. (2013). Activated ClpP kills persists and eradicates a chronic biofilm infection. *Nature*. 503. pg. 365-70. http://www.nature.com/nature/journal/v503/n7476/full/nature12790.html

- "Chronic infections are difficult to treat with antibiotics but are caused primarily by drug-sensitive pathogens. Dormant persister cells that are tolerant to killing by antibiotics are responsible for this apparent paradox."
- "Persisters are phenotypic variants of normal cells and pathways leading to dormancy are redundant, making it challenging to develop anti-persister compounds."
- "Biofilms shield persisters from the immune system, suggesting that an antibiotic for treating a chronic infection should be able to eradicate the infection on its own. We reasoned that a compound capable of corrupting a target in dormant cells will kill persisters. The acyldepsipeptide antibiotic (ADEP4) has been shown to activate the ClpP protease, resulting in death of growing cells. Here we show that ADEP4-activated ClpP becomes a fairly nonspecific protease and kills persisters by degrading over 400 proteins, forcing cells to self-digest."
- "Null mutants of ClpP arise with high probability, but combining ADEP4 with rifampicin produced complete eradication of Staphylococcus aureus biofilms in vitro and in a mouse model of a chronic infection.
- "Our findings indicate a general principle for killing dormant cells—activation and corruption of a target, rather than conventional inhibition. Eradication of a biofilm in an animal model by activating a protease suggests a realistic path towards developing therapies to treat chronic infections."

Consumer Reports. (June 2013). Consumer Reports investigation: Talking turkey. *Consumer Reports Magazine*. http://www.consumerreports.org/cro/magazine/2013/06/consumer-reports-investigation-talking-turkey/index.htm

- "In our first-ever lab analysis of ground turkey bought at retail stores nationwide, more than half of the packages of raw ground meat and patties tested positive for fecal bacteria. Some samples harbored other germs, including salmonella and staphylococcus aureus, two of the leading causes of foodborne illness in the U.S. Overall, 90 percent of the samples had one or more of the five bacteria for which we tested."

Consumer Reports. (February 2014). The high cost of cheap chicken. *Consumer Reports*. http://www.consumerreports.org/content/cro/en/consumer-reports-magazine/z2014/February/theHighCostOfCheapChicken.print.html

- "When you shop at your favorite grocery store, you probably assume that the food on display is safe to take home. But in the poultry aisle, that simple assumption could make you very sick. Consumer Reports' recent analysis of more than 300 raw chicken breasts purchased at stores across the U.S. found potentially harmful bacteria lurking in almost all of the chicken, including organic brands. In fact, we were conducting our research when news of the national salmonella outbreak linked to three Foster Farms chicken plants became public. In that case 389 people were infected, and 40 percent of them were hospitalized, double the usual percentage in most outbreaks linked to salmonella. (Read about sustainable alternatives when it comes to raising chickens and watch our video on the use of antibiotics in animals.)"

Courtney, C. M., Goodman, S. M., McDaniel, J. A., et al. (2015). Photoexcited quantum dots for killing multidrug-resistant bacteria. *Nature Materials.* www.nature.com/nmat/journal/vaop/ncurrent/full/nmat4542.html

- "Photoexcited quantum dots (QDs) can kill a wide range of multidrug-resistant bacterial clinical isolates, including methicillin-resistant *Staphylococcus aureus*."
- Nanotechnology including the use of quantum dots may be the one helpful hi-tech solution to the looming anti-microbial crisis, but only in selected health care institution.

Dantas, G., Sommer, M. O. A., Oluwasegun, R. D. and Church, G. M. (2008). Bacteria subsisting on antibiotics. *Science.* 320. pg. 100-103. http://arep.med.harvard.edu/pdf/Dantas08.pdf

- "Bacteria subsisting on antibiotics are surprisingly phylogenetically diverse, and many are closely related to human pathogens."
- "In addition to the finding that bacteria subsisting on natural and synthetic antibiotics are widely distributed in the environment, these results highlight an unrecognized reservoir of multiple antibiotic-resistance machinery. Bacteria subsisting on antibiotics are phylogenetically diverse and include many organisms closely related to clinically relevant pathogens. It is thus possible that pathogens could obtain antibiotic-resistance genes from environmentally distributed super-resistant microbes subsisting on antibiotics."

Davies, J. and Davies, D. (2010). Origins and evolution of antibiotic resistance. *Microbiology and Molecular Biology Reviews.* 74(3). pg. 417-33. http://mmbr.asm.org/content/74/3/417.full

- "Many resolutions and recommendations have been propounded, and numerous reports have been written, but to no avail: the development of antibiotic resistance is relentless."
- "Antibiotics have revolutionized medicine in many respects, and countless lives have been saved; their discovery was a turning point in human history. Regrettably, the use of these wonder drugs has been accompanied by the rapid appearance of resistant strains."
- "Stricter measures in infection control and antibiotic use [include] efforts to prevent dumping of antibiotics into the environment through sewer systems complete destruction of antibiotics before disposal should be common practice."
- "The tragedy is that most pharmaceutical companies are now shirking the responsibilities of their own business missions. The onus is on academia to furnish information on the multifunctional aspects of microbial network interactions that will provide the discovery tools of the future."

Davis, M. F. and Rutkow, L. (2012). 327 Regulatory strategies to combat antimicrobial resistance of animal origin: Recommendations for a science-based U.S. approach. *Tulane Environmental Law Journal.* 25(327). pg. 1-55. http://www.jhsph.edu/research/centers-and-institutes/johns-hopkins-center-for-a-livable-future/_pdf/research/clf_reports/Davis%20Regulatory%20Strategies.pdf

- "This article presents an update pertaining to nontherapeutic use of antimicrobials in livestock and to surveillance of antimicrobial-resistant pathogens of food animal origin."

D'Costa, V. M., McGrann, K. M., Hughes, D. W. and Wright, G. D. (2006). Sampling the antibiotic resistome. *Science.* 311(5759). pg. 374-7. http://www.ncbi.nlm.nih.gov/pubmed/16424339

- "Microbial resistance to antibiotics currently spans all known classes of natural and synthetic compounds. It has not only hindered our treatment of infections but also dramatically reshaped drug discovery, yet its origins have not been systematically studied. Soil-dwelling bacteria produce and encounter a myriad of antibiotics, evolving corresponding sensing and evading strategies. They are a reservoir of resistance determinants that can be mobilized into the microbial community. Study of this reservoir could provide an early warning system for future clinically relevant antibiotic resistance mechanisms."

Dellavalle, Curt. (2016). *The pollution in people: Cancer-causing chemicals in American's bodies.* Environmental Working Group. http://static.ewg.org/reports/2016/cancer_main/the-pollution-in-people/EWG_Cancer_Bio-Monitoring_Report_C02-pages.pdf?_ga=1.248454977.73987476.1464276744

Domenech, B., Munoz, M., Muraviev, D. N. and Macanas, J. (2013). Polymer-Silver nanocomposites as antibacterial materials. *Microbiology.* 4(1). pg. 630-40. http://www.formatex.info/microbiology4/vol1/630-640.pdf

- "Silver (Ag) has long been known to exhibit a strong toxicity towards a wide range of microorganisms. Thanks to these broad-spectrum antimicrobial properties, silver has been extensively used for biomedical applications and other environmental disinfection processes for centuries."
- "Due to their unique properties, silver nanoparticles (AgNPs) represent a reasonable alternative for boosting the development of new bactericides. Because of their high surface area to volume ratio and their high active surface (with highly active facets), metal nanoparticles (MNPs) exhibit remarkable and outstanding properties, such as increased catalytic activity. Therefore, AgNPs could be more reactive and become more antimicrobiologically active than the bulk counterpart."
- "Applications such in clothing, respirators, household water filters, contraceptives, antibacterial sprays, cosmetics, detergents, dietary supplements, cutting boards, shoes, cell phones, laptop keyboards, and children's toys are typical products currently in the market that exploit the antimicrobial properties of silver nanomaterials."
- "Even if the use of of AgNPs seems to open a new window of possibilities in the development of new-age antibacterial agents, some environmental and health safety risks, sometimes referred as nanotoxicity must be intensively considered."
- "Taking into account the antimicrobial power of the Ag-nanocomposites, these materials could be used in the near future for the development of artificial organs, engineered tissues or medical instruments."
- This article contains an extensive historical overview of silver as an antibacterial agent.

Donlan, R. M. (2002). Biofilms: Microbial life on surfaces. *Emerging Infectious Diseases.* 8(9). pg. 881-90. http://wwwnc.cdc.gov/eid/article/8/9/pdfs/02-0063.pdf

- "Microorganisms attach to surfaces and develop biofilms. Biofilm-associated cells can be differentiated from their suspended counterparts by generation of an extracellular polymeric substance (EPS) matrix, reduced growth rates, and the up- and down-regulation of specific genes."

- "An established biofilm structures comprises microbial cells and EPS, has a defined architecture, and provides an optimal environment for the exchange of genetic material between cells."
- "Biofilms have great importance for public health because of their role in certain infectious diseases and importance in a variety of device-related infections."

Donskey, C. J., Chowdhry, T. K. and Hecker, M. T. (2015). Effect of antibiotic therapy on the density of vancomycin-resistant enterococci in the stool of colonized patients. *New England Journal of Medicine.* 343(26). pg. 1-16. http://www.nejm.org/doi/full/10.1056/NEJM200012283432604.

- "During treatment with 40 of 42 antianaerobic-antibiotic regimens (95 percent), high-density colonization with vancomycin-resistant enterococci was maintained…the density of colonization decreased after these regimens were discontinued."
- "For patients with vancomycin-resistant enterococci in stool, treatment with antianaerobic antibiotics promotes high-density colonization. Limiting the use of such agents in these patients may help decrease the spread of vancomycin-resistant enterococci."

Drlica, K. S. and Perlin, D. S. (2010). *Antibiotic resistance: Understanding and responding to an emerging crisis.* Pearson Education, Upper Saddle River, NJ.

- "Pathogenic bacteria have been evolving and spreading resistance to diverse classes of antibiotics. As a result, we risk losing our ability to control and treat infectious diseases."

Drudy, D., Mullane, N. R., Quinn, T., Wall, P. G. and Fanning, S. (2006). Enterobacter sakazakii: an emerging pathogen in powdered infant formula. *Food Safety.* 42(7). pg. 996-1002. http://cid.oxfordjournals.org/content/42/7/996.long

- "Enterobacter sakazakii represents a significant risk to the health of neonates. This bacterium is an emerging opportunistic pathogen that is associated with rare but life-threatening cases of meningitis, necrotizing enterocolitis, and sepsis in premature and full-term infants. Infants aged <28 days are considered to be most at risk."

Drury, B., Scott, J., Rosi-Marshall, E. and Kelly, J. (2013). Triclosan exposure increases triclosan resistance and influences taxonomic composition of benthic bacterial communities. *Environmental Science and Technology.* 47(15). pg. 8923-30. http://pubs.acs.org/doi/abs/10.1021/es401919k

- "Triclosan (TCS) is a broad-spectrum antimicrobial compound that is incorporated into numerous consumer products. TCS has been detected in aquatic ecosystems across the U.S., raising concern about its potential ecological effects. We conducted a field survey and an artificial stream experiment to assess effects of TCS on benthic bacterial communities. Field sampling indicated that TCS concentrations in stream sediments increased with degree of urbanization. There was significant correlation between sediment TCS concentration and the proportion of cultivable benthic bacteria that were resistant to TCS, demonstrating that the levels of TCS present in these streams was affecting the native communities. An artificial stream experiment confirmed that TCS exposure could trigger increases in TCS resistance within cultivable benthic bacteria, and pyrosequencing analysis indicated that TCS resulted in decreased benthic bacterial diversity and shifts in bacterial community composition. One notable change was a 6-fold increase in the relative abundance of cyanobacterial sequences and a dramatic die-off of algae within the artificial streams. Selection of cyanobacteria over algae could have significant implications for higher trophic levels within streams. Finally, there were no observed effects of TCS on bacterial abundance or respiration rates, suggesting that bacterial density and function were highly resilient to TCS exposure."

Dzidic, S., Suskovic, J. and Kos, B. (2008). Antibiotic resistance mechanisms in bacteria: biochemical and genetic aspects. *Food Technology Biotechnology.* 46(1). pg. 11-21. http://www.ftb.com.hr/index.php/archives/70-volume-46-issue-no-1/291

European Centre for Disease Prevention and Control. (2012). *Gonococcal antimicrobial susceptibility surveillance in Europe – 2010.* ECDC, Stockholm. http://ecdc.europa.eu/en/publications/Publications/1206-Gonococcal-AMR.pdf

European Centre for Disease Prevention and Control. (2012). *Response plan to control and manage the threat of multidrug-resistant gonorrhoea in Europe.* ECDC, Stockholm. http://ecdc.europa.eu/en/publications/Publications/1206-ECDC-MDR-gonorrhoea-response-plan.pdf

Fanatico, A., Owens, C. and Emmert, J. (2009). Organic poultry production in the United States: Broilers. *Journal of Applied Poultry Research.* 18. pg. 355-66. http://sd.appstate.edu/sites/sd.appstate.edu/files/organicpoultry.pdf

Feinman, S. E. (1998). Antibiotics in animal feed – drug resistance revisited. *American Society for Microbiology.* 64(1). pg. 24-30. http://www.asm.org/ccLibraryFiles/FILENAME/000000004443/Jan98FeinmanFeature.pdf

- "MDR coliforns occur at a high frequency in humans living in agricultural areas, especially among those engaged in livestock production and their families."
- "High counts of MDR *E. coli* also are found in poultry, commercial chicken meat, slaughterhouses, packing facilities, and in institutionally prepared servings of chicken, including food served in hospitals."

Fey, P., et al. (2000). Ceftriaxone-resistant salmonella infection acquired by a child from cattle. *The New England Journal of Medicine.* 44. pg. 1242-49. http://digitalcommons.unl.edu/cgi/viewcontent.cgi?article=1043&context=zoonoticspub

- "The emergence of resistance to anti-microbial agents within the salmonellae is a world-wide problem that has been associated with the use of antibiotics in livestock."
- "Of the estimated 1.4 million salmonella infections that occur each year in the United States, most are in children and the elderly and approximately 600 are fatal."
- "Antibiotic-resistant strains of salmonella in the United States evolve primarily in livestock…The ceftriaxone-resistant isolate from the child was indistinguishable from one of the isolates from cattle, which was also resistant to ceftriaxone. Both ceftriaxone-resistant isolates were resistant to 13 antimicrobial agents."

File, Jr., T. M. (2006). Clinical implications and treatment of multiresistant streptococcus pneumoniae pneumonia. *Clinical Microbiology and Infectious Diseases.* 12(Suppl. 3). pg. 31-41. http://www.clinicalmicrobiologyandinfection.com/article/S1198-743X(14)61320-3/pdf

- "*Streptococcus pneumoniae* is the leading bacterial cause of community-acquired respiratory tract infections…Since the 1990s there has been a significant increase in drug-resistant *Streptococcus pneumoniae* (DRSP) due in large part to increased use of antimicrobials."

Fink, Sheri. (2016). Drug shortages forcing hard decisions on rationing treatments. *The New York Times.* http://www.nytimes.com/2016/01/29/us/drug-shortages-forcing-hard-decisions-on-rationing-treatments.html

- "In recent years, shortages of all sorts of drugs--anesthetics, painkillers, antibiotics, cancer treatments--have become the new normal in American medicine."

- "The American Society of Health-System Pharmacists currently lists inadequate supplies of more than 150 drugs and therapeutics, for reasons ranging from manufacturing problems to federal safety crackdowns to drug makers abandoning low-profit products."

Fischbach, M. A. and Walsh, C. T. (2009). Antibiotics for emerging pathogens. *Science*. 325(5944). pg. 1089-93.
http://www.ncbi.nlm.nih.gov/pmc/articles/PMC2802854/

- "Historically, most antibiotics have come from a small set of molecular scaffolds whose functional lifetimes have been extended by generations of synthetic tailoring. The emergence of multidrug resistance among the latest generation of pathogens suggests that the discovery of new scaffolds should be a priority…Two factors exacerbate this supply problem by creating unique dis-incentives for antibiotic development. First, antibiotics are used in smaller quantities than other drugs…Antibiotics yield lower revenues than most drugs."
- "Promising approaches to scaffold discovery are emerging: they include mining underexplored microbial niches for natural products, designing screens that avoid rediscovering old scaffolds, and repurposing libraries of synthetic molecules for use as antibiotics…The use of a newly approved antibiotic may be restricted to the treatment of serious bacterial infections. The result is a quandary; Resistance is on the rise while antibiotic discovery and development are on the decline."

Fisher, et al. (2012). Emerging fungal threats to animal, plant and ecosystem health. *Nature*. 484. pg. 186-94.
https://nature.berkeley.edu/garbelotto/downloads/fisher2012.pdf

Food and Drug Administration. (2013). *Guidance for industry: New animal drugs and new animal drug combination products administered in or on medicated feed or drinking water of food-producing animals: Recommendations for drug sponsors for voluntarily aligning product use conditions with GFI #209.* Center for Veterinary Medicine, FDA, Rockville, MD.
http://www.fda.gov/downloads/AnimalVeterinary/GuidanceComplianceEnforcement/GuidanceforIndustry/UCM299624.pdf

Food and Drug Administration. (2014). *Summary report on antimicrobials sold or distributed for use in food producing animals*. FDA.
http://www.fda.gov/downloads/ForIndustry/UserFees/AnimalDrugUserFeeActADUFA/UCM416983.pdf

- "Section 105 of the Animal Drug User Fee Amendments of 2008 (ADUFA) (P.L. 110-316; 122 Stat. 3509) amended section 512 of the Federal Food, Drug, and Cosmetic Act ("the Act") [21 U.S.C. 360b] to require that sponsors of approved and conditionally approved applications for new animal drugs containing an antimicrobial active ingredient submit an annual report to the Food and Drug Administration (FDA) on the amount of each such ingredient in the drug that is sold or distributed for use in food-producing animals, including information on any distributor-labeled product. This legislation was enacted to assist FDA in its continuing analysis of the interactions (including antimicrobial resistance), efficacy, and safety of antimicrobials approved for use in both humans and food-producing animals."

- "This summary report includes sales and distribution data of antimicrobial drugs that are specifically approved for antibacterial uses or are known to have antibacterial properties."
- "Many antimicrobial animal drugs are approved and labeled for use in multiple species."

ANTIMICROBIAL DRUGS APPROVED FOR USE IN FOOD-PRODUCING ANIMALS[1]
ACTIVELY MARKETED IN 2012
DOMESTIC SALES AND DISTRIBUTION DATA
REPORTED BY MEDICAL IMPORTANCE AND DRUG CLASS

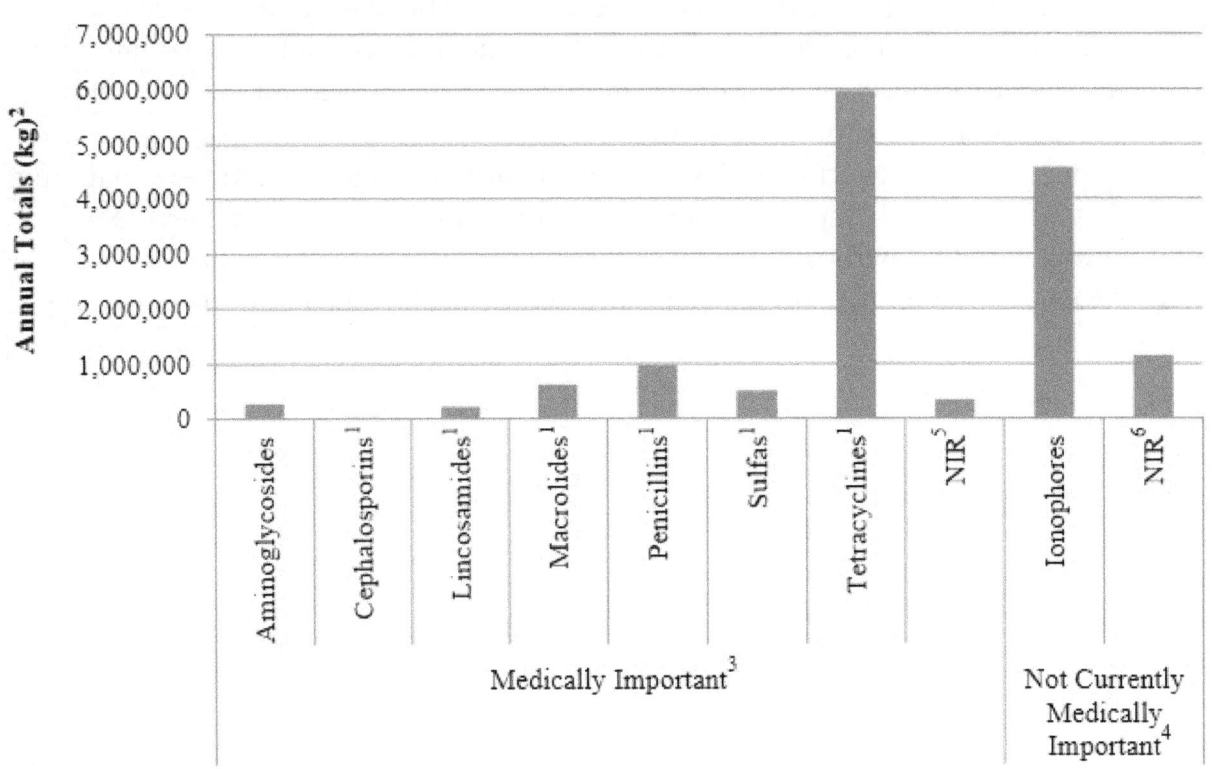

Medical Importance and Drug Class

Food and Drug Administration. (September 2, 2016). FDA issues final rule on safety and effectiveness of antibacterial soaps: Rule removes triclosan and triclocarban from over-the-counter antibacterial hand and body washes. *FDA News Release.* http://www.fda.gov/NewsEvents/Newsroom/PressAnnouncements/ucm517478.htm

Food and Water Watch and Beyond Pesticides. (2009). *Triclosan: What the research Shows.* Beyond Pesticides. http://www.beyondpesticides.org/antibacterial/triclosan-research-3-09.pdf

- "A growing list of household and personal care products are advertised as 'antibacterial' because they contain a chemical called triclosan. While the manufacturers of these products want you to think triclosan protects you from harmful bacteria, it turns out that it may be doing more harm than good."

Gale, E., Cundliffe, E., Reynolds, P., et al. (1981). *The molecular basis of antibiotic action*. John Wiley & Sons Ltd., New York, NY.

- The definitive survey of the action of antimicrobial drugs and the structure and biochemical activities of microorganisms.
- This was the first definitive study of the chemistry and structure of antibiotics by a well-known professor of chemical microbiology at the University of Cambridge who began his research in the late 1940s.

Gao, P., Nie, X., Zou, M., et al (2011). Recent advances in materials for extended-release antibiotic delivery system. *The Journal of Antibiotics*. 64. pg. 625-34.

- "By maintaining a constant plasma drug concentration over MIC for a prolonged period, extended-release dosage forms maximize the therapeutic effect of antibiotics while minimizing antibiotic resistance. Another undoubted advantage of extended-release formulation is improved patient compliance."
- "This review highlights the development of materials used in extended-release formulation and nanoparticles for antibiotic delivery."
- "Incomplete treatment may aggravate the development of antibiotic resistance. Many antibiotics have short half life values and need to be administered frequently, which also contributes to patient incompliance."
- "Until now, only few nanoparticle-based antimicrobial agents have been approved for clinical use. The limitation of their application is mainly caused by the high cost and unsatisfactory drug loading…[it is hoped that] 'nanoparticle-based' extended-release antibiotic delivery…will come to sight in the future."
- No mention of the future possibility of antibiotic winters.

Gardam, M. (2000). Is methicillin-resistant *Staphylococcus aureus* an emerging community pathogen? A review of the literature. *Canadian Journal of Infectious Disease and Medicine*. 11(4). pg. 202-11. http://www.ncbi.nlm.nih.gov/pmc/articles/PMC2094767/

- Yes, even by 2000 AD.
- "MRSA has emerged over the past 30 years to become a worldwide nosocomial pathogen and has recently been reported as a cause of community-acquired infections."
- "The changing epidemiology of MRSA is likely because of two mechanisms: the movement of nosocomial MRSA strains into the community and the de novo appearance of community strains resulting from the transfer of genetic material from methicillin-resistant Gram-positive organisms to sensitive *S aureus* strains."

- "The emergence of MRSA as a community pathogen has occurred at a slower rate than it did for penicillin-resistant *S aureus* (PRSA) in the 1950s and 1960s, possibly because the mechanism of methicillin resistance does not exhibit the same ease of transferability as that of penicillin resistance."
- "It appears, however, that MRSA strains of both nosocomial and community origin are now endemic in certain communities in different parts of the world. Few surveillance studies of non-hospitalized patient populations have been performed to date; thus, the true prevalence of MRSA in the community at large is essentially unknown."
- Another late 20th century preview of the upcoming 21st century antibiotic resistant pandemic.

Giedraitiene, A., Vitkauskiene, A., Naginiene, R. and Pavilonis, A. (2011). Antibiotic resistance mechanisms of clinically important bacteria. *Edicina (Kaunas)*. 47(3). pg. 137-46. http://www.ncbi.nlm.nih.gov/pubmed/21822035

- "Acquired resistance arises from: (i) mutations in cell genes (chromosomal mutation) leading to cross-resistance, (ii) gene transfer from one microorganism to other by plasmids (conjugation or transformation), transposons (conjugation), integrons and bacteriophages (transductions)."

Gilchrist, M., et al. (2007).The potential role of concentrated animal feeding operations in infectious disease epidemics and antibiotic resistance. *Environmental Health Perspectives*. 115(2). pg. 313-6. http://www.ncbi.nlm.nih.gov/pmc/articles/PMC1817683/

- "The industrialization of livestock production and the widespread use of nontherapeutic antimicrobial growth promotants has intensified the risk for the emergence of new, more virulent, or more resistant microorganisms. These have reduced the effectiveness of several classes of antibiotics for treating infections in humans and livestock."
- "[We] concurred with the World Health Organization call for a phasing-out of the use of antimicrobial growth promotants for livestock and fish production. We also agree that all therapeutic antimicrobial agents should be available only by prescription for human and veterinary use."
- "Concern about the risk of an influenza pandemic leads us to recommend that regulations be promulgated to restrict the co-location of swine and poultry concentrated animal feeding operations (CAFOs) on the same site and to set appropriate separation distances."

- "As the human population increases, and mega cities grow, there is greater risk that infectious diseases will evolve, emerge, or spread readily among the populace."
- "All segments of livestock production might potentially contribute to zoonotic disease, including transportation of livestock, manure handling practices, veterinary medicine, meat processing and animal rendering."
- Also see the CDC glossary, which includes terminology and definitions not included in this glossary, pgs. 107-11.

Gillis, Justin. (February 21, 2016). In Zika epidemic, a warning on climate change: Mosquitoes will thrive in a warming world. *The New York Times*. pg. 6, 9. http://www.nytimes.com/2016/02/21/world/americas/in-zika-epidemic-a-warning-on-climate-change.html

- "Over the coming decades, global warming is likely to increase the range and speed of the life cycle of the particular mosquitoes carrying these viruses, encouraging their spread deeper into temperate countries like the United States."
- "Already, climate change is suspected — though not proved — to have been a factor in a string of disease outbreaks afflicting both people and animals. These include the spread of malaria into the highlands of eastern Africa, the rising incidence of Lyme disease in North America, and the spread of a serious livestock ailment called bluetongue into parts of Europe that were once too cold for it to thrive."
- "The vihjruses [Zika and dengue] are being transmitted largely by the yellow fever mosquito, Aedes aegypti. That creature adapted long ago to live in human settlements, and developed a concomitant taste for human blood."

Gjessing, H. W. and Ruskin, R. (1977). Antibiotic activity of bacteria isolated from some Caribbean sponges. *Proceedings of the 12th meeting of the Association of Island Marine Laboratories of the Caribbean Curaivo (Netherlands Antilles)*. Association of the Institute of Marine Laboratories of the Caribbean. pg. 12-4.

Goossens, H., et al. (2005). Outpatient antibiotic use in Europe and association with resistance: A cross-national database study. *The Lancet*. 365. pg. 579-87. http://www.thelancet.com/journals/lancet/article/PIIS0140-6736(05)17907-0/abstract

- "Prescription of antibiotics in primary care in Europe varied greatly; the highest rate was in France (32:2 defined daily doses [DDD] per 1000 inhabitants daily) and the lowest was in the Netherlands (10-0 DDD per 1000 inhabitants daily)."
- "We noted a shift from the old narrow-spectrum antibiotics to the new broad-spectrum antibiotics."

- "We showed higher rates of antibiotic resistance in high consuming countries, probably related to the higher consumption in southern and eastern Europe than in northern Europe."

Gottlieb, T. and Nimmo, G. (2011). Antibiotic resistance is an emerging threat to public health: An urgent call to action at the Antimicrobial Resistance Summit 2011. *Medical Journal of Australia.* 194(6). pg. 281-3. https://www.asid.net.au/documents/item/139

- "A return to the 'pre-antibiotic era' would render many routine infections untreatable and would seriously affect current practice in surgery, intensive care, organ transplantation, neonatology and cancer services through major increases in morbidity and mortality. The time to act is now – before we lose these 'miracle' drugs for good."
- "The scourge of antimicrobial resistance has increased inexorably over the years. We believe that the window for overcoming antimicrobial resistance is still open, but we must act decisively now – Australia cannot bury its head in the sand any longer and hope that the problem will just go away."

Grady, Denise. (January 7th, 2015). New antibiotic stirs hope against resistant bacteria. *The New York Times.* http://www.nytimes.com/2015/01/08/health/from-a-pile-of-dirt-hope-for-a-powerful-new-antibiotic.html?_r=0

- "An unusual method for producing antibiotics may help solve an urgent global problem: the rise in infections that resist treatment with commonly used drugs, and the lack of new antibiotics to replace ones that no longer work. The method, which extracts drugs from bacteria that live in dirt, has yielded a powerful new antibiotic, researchers reported in the journal Nature on Wednesday."

Gu, B., Kelesidis, T., Tsiodras, et al. (2012). The emerging problem of linezolid-resistant Staphylococcus. *Journal of Antimicrobial Chemotherapy.* 68(1). pg. 4-11. http://jac.oxfordjournals.org/cgi/pmidlookup?view=long&pmid=22949625

Haack, S. K., Metge, D. W., Fogarty, L. R., et al. (2012). Effects on groundwater microbial communities of an engineered 30-day in situ exposure to the antibiotic sulfamethoxazole. *Environ. Sci. Technol.*46(14). pg. 7478-86. http://pubs.acs.org/doi/abs/10.1021/es3009776

- "Sulfamethoxazole (SMX) is one of the most frequently detected antibiotics in the environment."
- "Commonly detected concentrations of SMX in groundwater range up to $1.1 \mu gL^{-1}$."

- "Concentrations of antibiotics 2–3 orders of magnitude less than those used in clinical applications may influence ecological function through changes in community composition, and could promote antibiotic resistance through selection of naturally resistant bacteria."

Hammerum, A., Heuer, O., Emborg, H., et al. (2007). Danish integrated antimicrobial resistance monitoring and research program. *Emerging Infectious Disease*. 13. pg. 1632-9. http://www.ncbi.nlm.nih.gov/pmc/articles/PMC3375779/

Hammerum, A., Lester, C. and Heuer, O. (2010). Antimicrobial-resistant enterococci in animals and meat: A human health hazard*? Foodborne Pathogens and Disease*. 7. pg. 1137-46. http://www.ncbi.nlm.nih.gov/pubmed/20578915

Han, F., Lestari, S., Pu, S. and Ge, B. (2009). Prevalence and antimicrobial resistance among Campylobacter spp. in Louisiana retail chickens after the enrofloxacin ban. *Foodborne Pathogens and Disease*. 6. pg. 163-71. http://www.ncbi.nlm.nih.gov/pubmed/19099357

Harbath, S. and Samore, M. (2005). Antimicrobial resistance determinants and future control. *Emerging Infectious Diseases*. 11(6). pg. 794-801. http://www.ncbi.nlm.nih.gov/pmc/articles/PMC3367590/

- "At the beginning of the 21st century, antimicrobial resistance is common, has developed against every class of antimicrobial drug, and appears to be spreading into new clinical niches. We describe determinants likely to influence the future epidemiology and health impact of antimicrobial-resistant infections. Understanding these factors will ultimately optimize preventive strategies for an unpredictable future."

Table 1. Potential determinants influencing future dissemination and control of antimicrobial resistance

Dimension	Determinant	Potential control measures and interventions
Pathogen and microbial ecology	Evolution	Evolutionary engineering
	Survival fitness	Inhibition of microbial gene expression
	Virulence	Antibodies, antipathogenicity drugs, biologic response modifiers
	Commensal flora	Probiotics
	Laboratory detection and identification	Improved rapid diagnostic tests
Physician's prescribing practice	Antimicrobial drug usage pattern	Multimodal interventions
	Diversity of antimicrobial drug prescribing	Decision support tools
	Training and knowledge	Academic detailing and educational campaigns
Population characteristics	Migration, travel, and globalization	Screening and improved surveillance
	Case mix and host susceptibility to infections	Immunization; better control of chronic diseases
	Antimicrobial demand and health beliefs	Public information campaigns
	Transmission and infection rates	Hand hygiene and barrier precautions
Politics and healthcare policy	Healthcare policy	Change in reimbursement patterns
	Promotional activities by industry	Regulation
	Technologic development	New prevention and treatment approaches

- "These determinants can be grouped into 4 categories."

- "Whether the current epidemic of antimicrobial resistance is sustainable or will succumb to current efforts to limit its spread will be decided by an interaction of factors related to microorganisms, host, use patterns of antimicrobial drugs, and the impact of infection control measures and technologic development."
- "We hope that adding infection control and prudent use of antimicrobial agents to new drug development will avert the realization of pessimistic predictions about the future of antimicrobial resistance."
- Unfortunately, by early 2016, we are now facing a worldwide antibiotic resistance pandemic.

Hawkey, P. M. and Jones, A. M. (2009).The changing epidemiology of resistance. *Journal of Antimicrobial Chemotherapy.* 64(Suppl. 1). pg. i3-10. http://jac.oxfordjournals.org/content/64/suppl_1/i3.long

- "Resistance in Gram-positive bacteria is also widely distributed and increasing, with the emergence of community-associated methicillin-resistant *Staphylococcus aureus* (MRSA) blurring the distinction between hospital and community strains."
- "Surveillance data reported high levels of ESBL-producing strains of *Klebsiella pneumoniae* and *E. coli* in Australasia, ranging from <10% in Australia and Japan to >30% in Singapore and China for *K. pneumoniae* and from ~11% in Singapore to 25% in China for *E. coli*. Subsequent analysis of strains from China identified CTX-M-14 as the dominant genotype, which has been found particularly in the Far East but has also spread worldwide."
- "Pressures, both clinical and commercial, to use antibiotics in both humans and animals, the global mobility of populations and food products, ensure that the spread of MDR bacterial clones and resistance genes will be a continuing phenomenon."

Heuer, O., Pedersen, K., Andersen, J. and Madsen, M. (2002). Vancomycin-resistant enterococci (VRE) in broiler flocks 5 years after the avoparcin ban. *Microbial Drug Resistance.* 8. pg. 133-8. http://www.ncbi.nlm.nih.gov/pubmed/12118518

Hoa, P. T. P., Managaki, S., Nakada, N., et al. (2011). Antibiotic contamination and occurrence of antibiotic-resistant bacteria in aquatic environments of northern Vietnam. *Science of the Total Environment.* (409). pg. 2894-901. https://www.researchgate.net/publication/51215513_Antibiotic_contamination_and_occurrence_of_antibiotic-resistant_bacteria_in_aquatic_environments_of_northern_Vietnam

- "Southeast Asian countries commonly apply an integrated recycling farm system called VAC (Vegetable Aquaculture and Caged animal). In the VAC environment, antibiotics are released from animal and human origins, which would cause antibiotic-resistant bacteria (ARB)."

Howard, C. R. and Fletcher, N. F. (2012). Emerging virus diseases: Can we ever expect the unexpected. *Emerging Microbes and Infections.* 1(e46). pg. 1-11. http://www.nature.com/emi/journal/v1/n12/full/emi201247a.html

- "With new examples occurring approximately one each year, the majority are viruses originating from an animal host."
- "Changes to local ecosystems that perturb the balance between pathogen and principal host species is one of the major drivers, together with increasing urbanization of mankind and changes in human behavior."
- "Capacity to identify and control emerging diseases remains limited in poorer regions where many of these diseases have their origin [including] arenaviruses, filoviruses and hantaviruses."

Huang, S., Septimus, E., Kleinman, K., et al. (2013). Targeted versus universal decolonization to prevent ICU infection. *The New England Journal of Medicine.* 368. pg. 2255-65. http://www.nejm.org/doi/full/10.1056/NEJMoa1207290

- "Both targeted decolonization and universal decolonization of patients in intensive care units (ICUs) are candidate strategies to prevent health care–associated infections, particularly those caused by methicillin-resistant Staphylococcus aureus (MRSA)."

Huttner, A., Harbarth, S., Carlet, J., et al. (2013). Antimicrobial resistance: A global view from the 2013 World Healthcare-Associated Infections Forum. *Antimicrobial Resistance and Infection Control.* 2(31). pg. 1-13. http://www.aricjournal.com/content/2/1/31

- "Antimicrobial resistance (AMR) is now a global threat. Its emergence rests on antimicrobial overuse in humans and food-producing animals; globalization and suboptimal infection control facilitate its spread."
- "Antimicrobial conservation/stewardship programs have seen some measure of success in reducing antimicrobial overuse in humans, but their reach is limited to acute-care settings in high-income countries."
- "Outside the European Union, there is scant or no oversight of antimicrobial administration to food-producing animals, while evidence mounts that this administration leads directly to resistant human infection."

- "Antimicrobials are a non-renewable and endangered resource."
- "Microbes that are antibiotic producers have always needed to be resistant to their own antibiotic…Microbes have globalized along with their hosts, while at the same time antimicrobial consumption by these hosts—both humans and animals—has exploded."
- This article contains an important summary of abstracts on antimicrobial resistance, use, emergence, and conservation.

Table 2. The ten most urgent priorities for action against the spread of antimicrobial resistance cited by participants of the 4th WHAI Forum

For policy-makers and health authorities	
1	Limit the use of antimicrobials in food-producing animals by banning non-therapeutic applications, including growth promotion and metaphylaxis
2	Establish and enforce regulations on sales of antimicrobials or use in human medicine, including prohibition of over-the-counter sales worldwide
3	Develop a detailed charter on antimicrobial conservation to be ratified and upheld by ministries of health worldwide
4	Develop coordinated and culturally sensitive awareness campaigns targeting the general public and imparting the importance of protecting antimicrobials as a limited and non-renewable resource
5	Rigorously support the improvement of sanitation systems to eliminate resistant microbes in wastewater; regularly provide education about fundamental practices such as hand hygiene to prevent the spread of infection
6	Together with the pharmaceutical industry, explore (1) incentives to stimulate research and fast-track development of novel antimicrobials and (2) new economic models that reconcile public health interests with industry profitability
For the human and veterinary healthcare communities	
7	Establish standardized, universal methods and metrics for surveillance of antimicrobial use and resistance development respectively
8	In medical and veterinary school curricula, require universal and detailed instruction in microbial resistance development and the prudent use of antimicrobials; for physicians and veterinarians in training, require on-the-job refresher courses
For the general public	
9	Include patients and other antimicrobial consumers in the development and implementation of action plans
For industry	
10	Continue to develop and advance point-of-care rapid diagnostic tests to avoid

	the prescription of antibiotics for viral infections and allow more targeted therapy.
Conclusion	

Antimicrobial resistance is a clear and present danger. Immediate and coordinated measures must be taken worldwide to safeguard remaining antimicrobials and facilitate the development of novel antimicrobials. Bans on nontherapeutic antimicrobial consumption in livestock must be effectively championed despite strong resistance from industrial sectors. Conservation programs must be further optimized and implemented in other, non-acute healthcare settings such as long-term-care facilities. Educational programs targeting both antimicrobial prescribers and consumers must be further developed and supported. The general public must continue to be made aware of the current scale of AMR's threat. International collaboration among researchers and policy-makers must solidify to effect lasting reductions in the spread of antimicrobial resistance.

Hydromantis, Inc. (2010). *Emerging substances of concern in biosolids: Concentrations and effects of treatment processes. Final Report – literature Review.* CCME Project #447-2009. Canadian Council of Ministers of the Environment, University of Waterloo and Trent University.
http://www.ccme.ca/files/Resources/waste/biosolids/pn_1448_biosolids_esoc_final_e.pdf

- "Wastewater treatment facilities (WWTF) across Canada generate residual wastewater solids (sewage sludge) that require treatment for safeguarding human health and the environment prior to their use or disposal."
- "In this report, the term biosolids is applied to a treated material produced from raw sludge by processes such as anaerobic and aerobic digestion, composting, thermal or air drying, and alkaline stabilization with additives such as lime or cement kiln dust."
- "These ESOCs (emerging substances of concern) include an array of pharmaceuticals, personal care products, brominated flame retardants and industrial contaminants (such as plasticizers and surfactants)."
- "The detection [of] ESOCs in biosolids does not automatically imply that there is a risk for human health or the environment associated with proper biosolids management."
- The major categories of substances identified for review in the literature include:
  - o Industrial chemicals (plasticizers, pesticides, perfluorinated organic compounds, solvents, etc)
  - o Alkylphenols and their ethoxylates

- o Brominated flame retardants
- o Hormones and sterols
- o Pharmaceuticals
- o Personal Care Products
- o Certain metals (arsenic, silver selenium, mercury, etc.)
- o Other (e.g. polyaromatic hydrocarbons, polychlorinated dioxins and furans)
- Tables 31 to 42 contain a detailed listing of antibiotics found in the biosolids of waste water treatment facilities (WWTF) across Canada. Carbamazepine, anti-depressants, psycho-stimulants and mood altering drugs are also included.
- This publication includes 93 tables and an extensive bibliography. Much of the information in this text is not available in the U.S. due to political restrictions (U.S. Congress) on what the USGS, EPS, and other governmental entities are allowed to report on micropollutants in the environment, including the current restrictions on reporting the other micropollutants in the Flint, Michigan water supply.

Infectious Diseases Society of America (IDSA). (2011). Combating antimicrobial resistance: policy recommendations to save lives. *Clinical Infectious Diseases*. 52(Suppl.5). pg. S397-28. http://cid.oxfordjournals.org/content/52/suppl_5/S397.full#ref-1

- "Seven decades of medical advances enabled by antibiotics are now seriously threatened by the convergence of relentlessly rising antibiotic resistance and the alarming and ongoing withdrawal of most major pharmaceutical companies from the antibiotic market."
- "Our ability to respond to national security threats (e.g., bioterrorism and pandemics) also is in serious jeopardy."
- "This policy paper summarizes the Infectious Diseases Society of America's (IDSA) recommendations about how best to address the synergistic crises of rising rates of antibiotic resistance and waning approvals of new antibiotics."
- "Specific recommendations for Congress related to legislative action and funding needs are summarized in Tables 1 and 2."
- Most of the funding request and policy recommendations in this report have not been adopted.
- The comprehensive bibliography includes 129 citations.

Ismail, S., Perni, S., Pratten, J., et al. (2011). Efficacy of a novel light-activated antimicrobial coating for disinfecting hospital surfaces. *Infection Control and Hospital Epidemiology*. 32(11). pg. 1130-2. http://discovery.ucl.ac.uk/1326530/1/662377.pdf
54

Jelić, A., Gros, M., Petrović, M. et al. (2012). Occurrence and elimination of pharmaceuticals during conventional wastewater treatment. In: *Emerging and priority pollutants in rivers: Bringing science into river management plans.* Springer-Verlag, Berlin, Germany. http://www.springer.com/978-3-642-25721-6.

- "Conventional systems that use an activated sludge process are still widely employed for wastewater treatment, mostly because they produce effluents that meet required quality standards (suitable for disposal or recycling purposes), at reasonable operating and maintenance costs. However, this type of treatment has been shown to have limited capability of removing pharmaceuticals from wastewater."

Jernberg, C., Lofmark, S., Edlund, C. and Jansson, J. (2010). Long-term impacts of antibiotic exposure on the human intestinal microbiota. *Microbiology*. 156. pg. 3216-23. http://www.microbiologyresearch.org/docserver/fulltext/micro/156/11/3216.pdf?expires=1454086793&id=id&accname=guest&checksum=95A66B02321FF043FEB2A99ED5DAFD46

- "A disturbing consequence of antibiotic treatment has been the long-term persistence of antibiotic resistance genes, for example in the human gut. These data warrant use of prudence in the administration of antibiotics that could aggravate the growing battle with emerging antibiotic-resistant pathogenic strains."
- "Increasing antimicrobial resistance is a growing threat to human health and is mainly a consequence of excessive use of antimicrobial agents in clinical medicine."
- "It is important to also consider the role of the enormously diverse human commensal microbiota. It is generally acknowledged that the use of antibiotics causes selection for and enrichment of antimicrobial resistance, but it has also been believed until recently that the commensal microbiota is normalized a few weeks following withdrawl of the treatment."
- Also see Appendix 5: Commensals: Underappreciated Reservoirs of Antibiotic Resistance. (Marshall 2009)

Jones, K., Patel, N., Levy, M., et al. (2008). Global trends in emerging infectious diseases. *Nature*. 451. pg. 990-3. http://www.nature.com/nature/journal/v451/n7181/abs/nature06536.html

- "Colonization of in-dwelling catheters leads to biofilm formation and results in catheters serving as sources of continual infection in patients."

Jones A., Kuijper E. and Wilcox, M. (2013). Clostridium difficile: A European perspective. *Journal of Infectious Disease.* 66(2). pg. 115-28. http://www.ncbi.nlm.nih.gov/pubmed/23103666

- "Clostridium difficile infection is the leading cause of diarrhoea in the industrialised world. First identified in 1935, our knowledge about the clonal population structure, toxins and PCR ribotypes is still increasing. New PCR ribotypes and sequence types are frequently added. In the last decade hypervirulent strains have emerged and been associated with increased severity of disease, high recurrence and significant mortality."
- "Although previously a primarily hospital- or health-care acquired infection, since the 1990's C. difficile infections that are community-acquired have been increasingly reported. Risk factors include hospitalisation, advancing age and prior antibiotic use."
- "The ubiquitous presence of C. difficile in the environment and asymptomatic intestinal colonisation may be important reservoirs for infection and the changing epidemiology of C. difficile infection. Although surveillance in Europe is now a requirement of the European Commission, reporting is not standardised or mandatory. Here we review the current literature, guidelines on diagnosis and treatment and conclude by highlighting a number of areas where further research would increase our understanding."

Karpin, G. W., Morris, D. M., Ngo, M. T., et al. (2015). Transition metal diamine complexes with antimicrobial activity against staphylococcus aureus and methicillin-resistant S. aureus (MRSA). *Med. Chem. Commun.* 451. pg. 990-94. http://pubs.rsc.org/en/content/articlelanding/2015/md/c5md00228a#!divAbstract

- "Emerging infectious diseases (EIDs) are a significant burden on global economies and public health"
- "We find that 54.3% of EID events are caused by bacteria or rickettsia, reflecting a large number of drug-resistant microbes in our database."
- "Global resources to counter disease emergence are poorly allocated, with the majority of the scientific and surveillance effort focused on countries from where the next important EID is least likely to originate."

Kassotis, C. D., Tillit, D. E., Lin, C-H., et al. (2016). Endocrine-disrupting chemicals and oil and natural gas operations: Potential environmental contamination and recommendations to assess complex environmental mixtures. *Environ. Health Perspect.* 24(3). pg. 256-64. http://ehp.niehs.nih.gov/1409535/

Katz, J. (2004). Hand washing and hand disinfection: More than your mother taught you. *Anesthesiology Clinics of North America.* 22(3). pg. 115-28. http://www.sciencedirect.com/science/article/pii/S0889853704000276

Kesselheim, A. S. and Outterson, K. (2009). Fighting antibiotic resistance: Marrying new financial incentives to meeting public health goals. *Health Affairs.* 29(9). pg. 1689-96. http://content.healthaffairs.org/content/29/9/1689.full.pdf+html

- "We review a number of proposals intended to bolster drug development, including such financial incentives for pharmaceutical manufacturers as extending the effective patent life for new antibiotics. However, such strategies directly conflict with the clear need to reduce unnecessary antibiotic prescriptions and could actually increase prescription use."

Khachatourians, G. C. (1998). Agricultural use of antibiotics and the evolution and transfer of antibiotic-resistant bacteria. *Canadian Medical Association Journal.* 159(9). pg. 1129-36. http://www.ncbi.nlm.nih.gov/pmc/articles/PMC1229782/

- "Intensive animal production involves giving livestock animals large quantities of antibiotics to promote growth and prevent infection. These uses promote the selection of antibiotic resistance in bacterial populations. The resistant bacteria from agricultural environments may be transmitted to humans, in whom they cause disease that cannot be treated by conventional antibiotics."
- "Microbial resistance to antibiotics is on the rise, in part because of inappropriate use of antibiotics in human medicine but also because of practices in the agricultural industry."
- "The resistant bacteria from agricultural environments may be transmitted to humans, in whom they cause disease that cannot be treated by conventional antibiotics."
- This ancient publication (1998) contains interesting diagrams illustrating the development and movement of antibiotic resistance genes.

Khouse.org. (April 5, 2011). *Plastic nanoparticles fight MRSA.* eNews. http://www.khouse.org/enews_article/2011/1759/print/.

- "Engineers in San Jose, California have created a new form of antibiotic out of manmade nanoparticles…able to search out and destroy even the scariest of antibiotic-resistant bacteria. When their job of slaughtering the bacterial enemy is finished, the nanoparticles harmlessly biodegrade away."
- "The engineers have given the nanoparticles a charge so that they are attracted to oppositely charged bacteria. In this way, they can be used to target infected cells,

reportedly eradicating bacteria like MRSA while leaving beneficial bacteria alone."

- "Rather than attacking the bacterial DNA, these brutal plastic machetes beat down the cell walls, destroying the bacteria from the outside-in."
- " 'These are designed to slice the cell membrane, to rip the membrane up and eliminate the contents', explains James Hedrick, advanced organic materials scientist at IBM Almaden Research Center. 'It's kind of like the way a virus would work – a virus drills a pore, empties the contents and hijacks it. This is drilling in little holes, and all the contents leak out.'"
- "While the technology sounds promising, it has yet to be tested on humans. IBM declares that the nanoparticles harmlessly degrade into an innocuous byproduct…A great deal of testing needs to be done to make sure that the nanoparticles only attack the cells of the organisms they are intended to attack.
- The correct title for this article should be "Nanoplastic Particles" since this is a synthetic nanoparticle. Updates since 2011 seem elusive.

Kodjak, Alison. (September 2, 2016). FDA bans 19 chemicals used in antibacterial soaps. *NPR News.* http://www.npr.org/sections/health-shots/2016/09/02/492394717/fda-bans-19-chemicals-used-in-antibacterial-soaps

Kolpin, D., Furlong, E., Meyer, M., et al. (2002). Pharmaceuticals, hormones, and other organic wastewater contaminants in US Streams, 1999-2000; a national reconnaissance. *Environmental Science and Technology.* 36(6). pg. 1202-11. http://digitalcommons.unl.edu/cgi/viewcontent.cgi?article=1064&context=usgsstaffpub

Kostich, M. S. and Lazorchak, J. M. (2008). Risks to aquatic organisms posed by human pharmaceutical use. *Sci Total Environ.* 389(2-3). pg. 329-39. http://www.ncbi.nlm.nih.gov/pubmed/17936335

Kostich, M. S., Batt, A. L. and Lazorchak, J. M. (2014). Concentration of prioritized pharmaceuticals in effluents from 50 large wastewater treatment plants in the US and implications for risk estimation. *Environmental Pollution.* 184. Pg. 354-359. http://www.epa.gov/sites/production/files/2014-09/documents/50_large_wwtp_effluent.pdf

- "The primary route of APIs into surface waters is believed to be excretion by patients into wastewater collection systems…Over 1000 APIs are approved for use in the US…but most studies examining environmental occurrence only report concentrations of a handful of analytes."
- "Little or no measured concentration data are available for a number of widely prescribed APIs." (Kostich 2010)

- "Here we report the measured concentrations of 56 APIs and 7 API metabolites in effluent samples from fifty very large (15 to 660 MGD) wastewater treatment plants (WWTPs) located across the US."
- **"Antibiotic concentrations may inhibit the growth of some naturally occurring beneficial microbes, and may facilitate early steps in the acquisition of clinically significant resistance. These conclusions can be tentatively extended to all prescription pharmaceuticals in current use."**
- "In addition to direct toxicological risks, concern has been raised about the potential for antibiotic residues in wastewater giving rise to antibiotic resistant human pathogens." (Webb 2003)
- "Microbial sensitivity to antibiotics is typically expressed as the minimum inhibitory concentration (MIC) of the antibiotic, which is the lowest concentration of antibiotic, in a standard in vitro test system causing reliable inhibition of microbial growth."
- "Clinically significant antibiotic resistance is defined in terms of the concentrations of antibiotic that can be safely maintained in a target tissue in a patient without causing excessive adverse side-effects. This concentration is termed a 'breakpoint' concentration (BP)."
- "Microbes whose MIC is greater than the BP for a given antibiotic are considered to have clinically significant resistance to the antibiotic in question. One way to estimate the selective pressure for development of clinically significant antibiotic resistance is comparison of MECs to the MIC and BP (Webb 2003; Kostich 2008). The highest MEC to BP ratio we observed was 0.0003, for the antibiotic ofloxacin (maximum MEC = 600 ng/L, BP = 2 µg/mL, or 2 million ng/L), suggesting no real risk of direct selection of clinically significant resistance."
- "On the other hand, the highest MEC to MIC ratio, 0.66 was also for ofloxacin (MIC = 0.001 µg/mL), and the second highest ratio (0.26) was for ciprofloxacin (MIC = 0.001 µg/mL). Because these ratios are close to one, they suggest the possibility for growth inhibition of some naturally occurring (and potentially beneficial) bacteria, and perhaps for initial acquisition of low level antibiotic resistance by exposed pathogens, particularly if assuming a concentration addition model for mixtures of antibiotics with common modes of action."
- "Such low level antibiotic resistance would not be directly clinically relevant, but it may facilitate faster development of clinically significant resistance when further selection with higher concentrations of antibiotics is applied, for instance in a treated patient."

Krasilnokova, D. N. (1961). On antibiotic properties of microorganism isolated from various depths of the world oceans. *Microbiology*. 30. pg. 545-50.

Kube, M., Beck, A., Zinder, S. H., et al. (2005). Genome sequence of the chlorinated compound-respiring bacterium *Dehalococcoides* species strain CBDB1. *Nature Biotechnology*. 23(10). pg 1269-73.
http://www.nature.com/nbt/journal/v23/n10/full/nbt1131.html

- "*Dehalococcoides* species are strictly anaerobic bacteria, which catabolize many of the most toxic and persistent chlorinated aromatics and aliphatics by reductive dechlorination and are used for *in situ* bioremediation of contaminated sites."

Kumar, S., et al. (2013). Antimicrobial resistance in India: A review. *Journal of Natural Science, Biology and Medicine*. 4(2). pg. 286-91.
http://www.ncbi.nlm.nih.gov/pmc/articles/PMC3783766/

- "There is an urgent need to develop and strengthen antimicrobial policy, standard treatment guidelines, national plan for containment of AMR and research related to public health aspects of AMR at community and hospital level in India."

Kuster, A., et al. (2014). Pharmaceuticals in the environment: Scientific evidence of risks and its regulation. *Philosophical Transactions of the Royal Society*. 369(1656). pg. 479-85. http://rstb.royalsocietypublishing.org/content/369/1656/20130587

- "10% of pharmaceutical products are of note regarding their potential environmental risk...for human medicinal products, hormones, **antibiotics**, analgesics, antidepressants and antineoplastics indicated an environmental risk...For veterinary products, hormones, antibiotics and parasiticides were most often discussed as being environmentally relevant"

Lakeslee, S. (February 2, 2016). Post-cesarean bacteria transfer could change health for life, study shows. *The New York Times*. pg. A-21.

- "The first germs to colonize a newborn delivered vaginally come almost exclusively from the mother. But the first to reach an infant born by cesarean section come mostly from the environment – particularly bacteria from inaccessible or less-scrubbed areas like lamps and walls, and from skin cells from everyone else in the delivery room."
- "Some epidemiological studies have suggested that C-section babies may have an elevated risk for developing immune and metabolic disorders, including Type 1 diabetes, allergies, asthma and obesity."

- "Scientists have theorized that these children may be missing key bacteria known to play a large role in shaping the immune system from the moment of birth onward."

Lebedeva, M. N. and Markianovic, E. M. (1971). Antibiotic features of heterotrophic bacteria in southern seas. *Proceedings of the 55th International Colloquium of Medical Oceanography*. pg. 335-52.

Lemos, M. L., Toranzo, A. and Barja, J. L. (1985). Antibiotic activity of epiphytic bacteria isolated from intertidal seaweeds. *Microbial Ecology*. 11. pg. 149-64. http://www.ncbi.nlm.nih.gov/pubmed/24221303

Levy, S. (1998). Multidrug resistance-a sign of the times. *New England Journal of Medicine*. 338. pg. 1376-8. http://www.ncbi.nlm.nih.gov/pubmed/9571260

Levy, S. (2001). Antibiotic resistance: consequences of inaction. *Clinical Infectious Diseases*. 33 (Supplement 3). pg. S124-29. http://cid.oxfordjournals.org/content/33/Supplement_3/S124.full

- "An emerging problem has grown to a crisis. Resistance is an ecological phenomenon stemming from the response of bacteria to the widespread use of antibiotics and their presence in the environment."

Levy, S. B. (2002). Factors impacting on the problem of antibiotic resistance. *Journal of Antimicrobial Chemotherapy*. (49). pg. 25-30.

- "Besides antibiotics, there is the mounting use of other agents aimed at destroying bacteria, namely the surface antibacterials now available in many household products. These too enter the environment. The stage is thus set for an altered microbial ecology."
- "In order to curb the resistance problem, we must encourage the return of the susceptible commensal flora. They are our best allies in reversing antibiotic resistance."
- "Confronted by increasing amounts of antibiotics over the past 60 years, bacteria have responded to the deluge with the propagation of progeny no longer susceptible to them."
- "Antibiotic residues can be found in the environment for long periods of time after treatment."

Levy, S. and Marshall, B. (2004). Antibacterial resistance worldwide: Causes, challenges and responses. *Nature Medicine Supplement* 10(12). pg. S122-9. http://www.nature.com/nm/journal/v10/n12s/abs/nm1145.html

- "Today, clinically important bacteria are characterized not only by single drug resistance but by multiple antibiotic resistance – the legacy of past decades of antimicrobial use and misuse."

Li, J., Nation, R. L., Milne, R. W. et al. (2005). Evaluation of colistin as an agent against multi-resistant Gram-negative bacteria. *International Journal of Antimicrobial Agents*. pg. 11-25. http://www.ijaaonline.com/article/S0924-8579(04)00365-6/pdf

- "The widespread resistance of microorganisms to antibiotics threatens to be a future medical diaster."
- "Infections caused by multi-resistant Gram-negative bacteria, particularly *Pseudomonas aeruginosa*, are incrasing worldwide. In patients with cystic fibrosis (CF), resistance in *P. aeruginosa* to numerous anti-pseudomonal agents is becoming common…It is likely that colistin will be an important antimicrobial option against multi-resistant Gram-negative bacteria, for some years to come."
- Not so many years as the medical community would have liked.

Li, J. and Vederas, J. (2009). Drug discovery and natural products: End of an era or an endless frontier? *Science*. 325(5937). pg. 161-5. http://www.ncbi.nlm.nih.gov/pubmed/19589993

- "Pharmaceutical research expanded after the Second World War to include massive screening of microorganisms for new antibiotics because of the discovery of penicillin. By 1990, about 80% of drugs were either natural products or analogs inspired by them."
- "Antibiotics (e.g., penicillin, tetracycline, erythromycin), antiparasitics (e.g., avermectin), antimalarials (e.g., quinine, artemisinin), lipid control agents (e.g., lovastatin and analogs), immunosuppresants for organ transplants (e.g., cyclosporine, rapamycins) and anticancer drugs (e.g., taxol, doxorubicin) revolutionized medicine."
- "Life expectancy in much of the world lengthened from about 40 years early in the 20th century to more than 77 years today [2008]."
- "Many pharmaceutical firms have eliminated their natural product research in the past decade…Is the era of discovery of new drugs from natural sources ending?"
- "Although the current industry model for drug discovery does not favor natural products, the resource is so vast as to seem unlimited, and these emerging tools will provide exhilarating discoveries leading to new medicines."

Li, X. and Nikaido, H. (2009). Efflux-medicated drug resistance in bacteria: An update. *National Institute of Health.* 69(12). pg. 1555-623. http://www.ncbi.nlm.nih.gov/pmc/articles/PMC2847397/

- "Drug efflux pumps play a key role in drug resistance and also serve other functions in bacteria…These pumps are mostly encoded on the chromosome although they can also be plasmid-encoded…In the past five years, significant progress has been achieved in further understanding of drug resistance-related efflux transporters."

Ling, L., Schneider, T., Peoples, A., et al. (2015). A new antibiotic kills pathogens without detectable resistance. *Nature.* 517. Pg. 455-9. http://www.nature.com/articles/nature14098.epdf?referrer_access_token=7qgWoiQWA kWIZtd4FOUq09RgN0jAjWel9jnR3ZoTv0PvwA6rMMnycnymQk5ZOpb5ktLjj6cTh7 j_4Otw8h3aTDBBDNFm-oDdcgGAruW1Qh8em_qgL58a0PI3KtqoXynG

- "Uncultured bacteria make up approximately 99% of all species in external environments, and are an untapped source of new antibiotics."
- "We developed…a new antibiotic that we term teixobactin, discovered in a screen of uncultured bacteria. Teixobactin inhibits cell wall synthesis by binding to a highly conserved motif of lipid II (precursor of peptidoglycan) and lipid III (precursor of cell wall teichoic acid)."
- "Here we report a new antibiotic that we term teixobactin, discovered in a screen of uncultured bacteria."
- "We did not obtain any mutants of Staphylococcus aureus or Mycobacterium tuberculosis resistant to teixobactin. The properties of this compound suggest a path towards developing antibiotics that are likely to avoid development of resistance."

Livermore, D. M., Canton, R., Gniadkowski, M., et al. (2007). CTX-M: Changing the face of ESBLs in Europe. *Journal of Antimicrobial Chemotherapy.* 59. pg. 165-74. http://jac.oxfordjournals.org/content/59/2/165.full

- "Since around 2000—earlier in Poland and Spain and later in France and the UK—dramatic shifts have occurred in the prevalence and types of extended- β-lactamases (ESBLs) in Europe."
- "Subsequently, CTX-M ESBLs have become dominant, with many infections in 'complicated community' patients, usually with underlying disease, recent antibiotic usage, or healthcare contact."

- "Irrespective of the particular enzyme, most producers are multiresistant. These changing patterns present major therapeutic and infection control challenges, with the public health intervention points unclear."
- "It is clear that Europe is moving to a situation where ESBLs are more common and less confined to hospitals, as well as one where *E. coli* is a major host species. If so, the opportunities for control are disturbingly small."

Loffler, C., Bohmer, F., Hornumg, A., et al. (2014). Dental care resistance prevention and antibiotic prescribing modification – the cluster-randomised controlled DREAM trial. *Implementation Science.* 9(27). pg. 1-66.
http://www.ncbi.nlm.nih.gov/pmc/articles/PMC3936853/

- "In Europe, dentistry accounts for a comparatively high amount of antibiotic prescriptions."
- "We expect the results of this trial to have a major impact on antibiotic prescription strategies and practices in Germany."

Lubick, N. (2011). Antibiotic resistance shows up in India's drinking water. *Nature.* Nature/doi:10.1038/news.2011.218.

- "Bacteria carrying a gene that confers resistance to a major class of antibiotics have shown up in samples of drinking water and sewage seepage from New Delhi, researchers report in The Lancet Infectious Diseases today…This is the first report to find NDM-1 in environmental samples unconnected to hospitals or infected patients…across New Delhi, a city with 21 million inhabitants."
- "In terms of resistance, the part of the iceberg that's important is what we don't see in hospitals-and in India, that part is absolutely massive."

Magiorakos, A.-P., Srinivasan, A., Carey, R. B., et al. (2012). Multidrug-resistant, extensively drug-resistant and pandrug-resistant bacteria: an international expert proposal for interim standard definitions for acquired resistance. *European Society of Clinical Microbiology and Infectious Diseases.* (18). pg. 268-81.
http://www.clinicalmicrobiologyandinfection.com/article/S1198-743X(14)61632-3/pdf

- "Many different definitions for multidrug-resistant (MDR), extensively drug-resistant (XDR) and pandrug-resistant (PDR) bacteria are being used in the medical literature to characterize the different patterns of resistance found in healthcare-associated, antimicrobial-resistant bacteria."
- "A group of international experts came together through a joint initiative by the European Centre for Disease Prevention and Control (ECDC) and the Centers for Disease Control and Prevention (CDC), to create a standardized international terminology with which to describe acquired resistance profiles."

- "MDR was defined as acquired non0susceptibility to at least one agent in three or more antimicrobial categories, XDR was defined as non-susceptibility to at least one agent in all but two or fewer antimicrobial categories (i.e. bacterial isolates remain susceptible to only one or two categories) and PDR was defined as non-susceptibility to all agents in all antimicrobial categories."

Marshall, Bonnie, Ochieng, Dorothy, and Levy, Stuart. (2009). Commensals: Underappreciated reservoir of antibiotic resistance. *Microbe*. 4(5). Pg. 231-238. http://www.asm.org/ccLibraryFiles/FILENAME/000000004865/znw005092945p.pdf

Marston, H. D., Dixon, D. M., Knisely, J. M., et al. (2016). Antimicrobial resistance. *JAMA*. 316(11). pg.1193-204. http://jama.jamanetwork.com/article.aspx?articleid=2553454

Martinez, J. L. (2008). Antibiotics and antibiotic resistance genes in natural environments. *Science*. 321(5887). pg. 365-7. http://www.ncbi.nlm.nih.gov/pubmed/18635792

Martinez, J. L. (2009). Environmental pollution by antibiotics and by antibiotic resistance determinants. *Environmental Pollution*. 157(11). pg. 2893-902. http://www.ncbi.nlm.nih.gov/pubmed/19560847

- "Antibiotics are extensively used for animal farming and for agricultural purposes. Residues from human environments and from farms may contain antibiotics and antibiotic resistance genes that can contaminate natural environments."
- "The clearest consequence of antibiotic release in natural environments is the selection of resistant bacteria. The same resistance genes found at clinical settings are currently disseminated among pristine ecosystems without any record of antibiotic contamination."
- "Nevertheless, the effect of antibiotics on the biosphere is wider than this and can impact the structure and activity of environmental microbiota."

Martinez, J. L. (2012). Natural antibiotic resistance and contamination by antibiotic resistance determinants: The two ages in the evolution of resistance to antimicrobials. *Frontiers in Microbiology*. 3. pg. 1. http://www.ncbi.nlm.nih.gov/pmc/articles/PMC3257838/

Masse, D. I., Cata Saady, N. M. and Gilbert, Y. (2014). Potential of biological processes to eliminate antibiotics in livestock manure: An overview. *Animals*. 4. pg. 146-163. http://www.mdpi.com/2076-2615/4/2/146/pdf

- "Beside their use to treat infections, antibiotics are used excessively as growth promoting factors in livestock industry. Animals discharge in their feces and urine between 70% - 90% of the antibiotic administrated unchanged or in active metabolites. Because livestock manure is re-applied to land as a fertilizer, concerns are growing over spread of antibiotics in water and soil."
- Anaerobic digestion [has the potential] to degrade antibiotics in livestock manure."

Mathur, S. and Singh, R. (2005). Antibiotic resistance in food lactic acid bacteria-a review. *International Journal of Food Microbiology*. 105(3). pg. 281-95.

- "Many investigators have speculated that commensal bacteria including lactic acid bacteria (LAB) may act as reservoirs of antibiotic resistance genes similar to those found in human pathogens. The main threat associated with these bacteria is that they can transfer resistance genes to pathogenic bacteria."
- "Distinction between intrinsic and acquired resistance is difficult as it is not possible to trace an investigated strain into the preantibiotic era."
- "There is no barrier between pathogenic (e.g. streptococci), potentially pathogenic (e.g. enterococci) and commensal (e.g. enteric lactobacilli, lactococci) LAB regarding acquired resistances."
- "LAB, like all other bacteria are prone to gene exchange to enhance survival in antibiotic containing environments."

Mauldin, P. D., Salgado, C. D., Hansen, I. S., et al. (2010). Attributable hospital cost and length of stay associated with health care-associated infections caused by antibiotic-resistant gram-negative bacteria. *Antimicrobial Agents and Chemotherapy*. 54(1). pg. 109-115. http://www.ncbi.nlm.nih.gov/pmc/articles/PMC2798544/

- "The objective of the present study was to determine the additional total hospital cost and LOS attributable to health care-associated infections (HAIs) caused by antibiotic-resistant, gram-negative (GN) pathogens."

McArthur, J. V., Tuckfield, R. C., Lindell, A. H. and Baker-Austin, C. (2011). When rivers become reservoirs of antibiotic resistance: Industrial effluents and gene nurseries. *Proceedings of the 2011 Georgia Water Resources Conference, held April 11-13, 2011 at the University of Georgia.* https://smartech.gatech.edu/bitstream/handle/1853/46105/4.5.1McArthur.pdf

- "Some water resources have become reservoirs af antibiotic resistance genes that can, under natural conditions, be transferred to water-borne pathogens."

66

- "The current opinion in the scientific community is that the rapid and continuing increase in antibiotic resistance found in clinical settings is caused by the misuse and overuse of antibiotics in medicine and agriculture."
- "Bacteria exposed to heavy metal pollution show elevated levels of antibiotic resistance (AR) and multiple antibiotic resistance (MAR) without ever being directly exposed to antibiotics."

McBryde, E., Bradley, L., Whitby, M. and McElwain, D. (2004). An investigation of contact transmission of methicillin-resistant Staphylococcus aureus. *Journal of Hospital Infection.* 58(2). pg. 104-108. http://www.journalofhospitalinfection.com/article/S0195-6701(04)00251-8/abstract

- "Hand hygiene is critical in the healthcare setting and it is believed that methicillin-resistant Staphylococcus aureus (MRSA), for example, is transmitted from patient to patient largely via the hands of health professionals. A study has been carried out at a large teaching hospital to estimate how often the gloves of a healthcare worker are contaminated with MRSA after contact with a colonized patient. The effectiveness of handwashing procedures to decontaminate the health professionals' hands was also investigated, together with how well different healthcare professional groups complied with handwashing procedures. The study showed that about 17% (9–25%) of contacts between a healthcare worker and a MRSA-colonized patient results in transmission of MRSA from a patient to the gloves of a healthcare worker. Different health professional groups have different rates of compliance with infection control procedures. Non-contact staff (cleaners, food services) had the shortest handwashing times. In this study, glove use compliance rates were 75% or above in all healthcare worker groups except doctors whose compliance was only 27%."

McDonald, M. and Blondeau, J. M. (2010). Emerging antibiotic resistance in ocular infections and the role of fluoroquinolones. *Journal of Cataract Refractive Surgery.* 36(9). pg. 1588-98. http://www.ncbi.nlm.nih.gov/pubmed/20692574

- "A growing body of evidence implicates environmental organisms as reservoirs of these resistance genes…We report a screen of a sample of the culturable microbiome of Lechuguilla Cave, New Mexico. In a region of the cave that has been isolated for over 4 million years…some strains were resistant to 14 different commercially available antibiotics."
- "The prevalence of resistance, even in microbiomes isolated from human use of antibiotics…supports a growing understanding that antibiotic resistance is natural, ancient, and hard wired in the microbial pangenome."

McKenna, M. (2013). Antibiotic resistance: The last resort. *Nature*. 499. pg. 394-96.

- "Health officials are watching in horror as bacteria become resistant to powerful carbapenem antibiotics-one of the last drugs on the shelf."
- "One of the reasons why the resistant strains spread so rapidly was that they were difficult to detect."

McNeil, D. G. (January 14, 2016). Virus in South America may bring C.D.C. alert. *The New York Times*. pg. A13. http://www.nytimes.com/2016/01/16/health/zika-virus-cdc-pregnant-women-travel-warning.html?_r=0

- "Federal health officials on Friday advised pregnant women to postpone traveling to 13 Latin American or Caribbean countries and Puerto Rico where mosquitoes are spreading the Zika virus, which has been linked to brain damage in babies."
- "Women considering becoming pregnant were advised to consult doctors before traveling to countries with Zika cases, and all travelers were urged to avoid mosquito bites, as were residents of Puerto Rico and the United States Virgin Islands."
- "Zika virus has been found in brain tissue and amniotic fluid from babies who died in the womb or were born with microcephaly."
- "The virus first appeared on the South American continent in May."
- "The C.D.C. advisory applies to 14 Western Hemisphere countries and territories: Brazil, Colombia, El Salvador, French Guiana, Guatemala, Haiti, Honduras, Martinique, Mexico, Panama, Paraguay, Suriname, Venezuela, and the Commonwealth of Puerto Rico."
- "More than a dozen isolated cases of Zika infection have been found in the continental United States."

McNeil, D. G. (February, 23, 2016). The potential hidden toll of Zika: Infants may later have mental health issues. *The New York Times*. pg. D1, D5. http://www.nytimes.com/2016/02/23/health/zika-may-increase-risk-of-mental-illness-researchers-say.html

- "Even infants who appear normal at birth may be at higher risk for mental illnesses later in life if their mothers were infected during pregnancy, many researchers fear."
- "The Zika virus, they say, closely resembles some infectious agents that have been linked to the development of autism, bipolar disorder and schizophrenia."

McNeill, R., Nelson, D. J. and Abutaleb, Y. (September 7, 2016). 'Superbug' scourge spreads as U.S. fails to track rising human toll. *Reuters*. http://www.reuters.com/investigates/special-report/usa-uncounted-surveillance/

Mellon, M., Benbrook, C. and Benbrook, K. (2001). *Hogging It: Estimates of antimicrobial abuse in livestock.* Union of Concerned Scientists, Cambridge, MA. http://www.iatp.org/files/Hogging_It_Estimates_of_Antimicrobial_Abuse_in.pdf

Menichetti, F. (2005). Current and emerging serious Gram-positive infections. *Clinical Microbiology Infections.* 11(Suppl. 3). pg. 22-28. http://www.clinicalmicrobiologyandinfection.com/article/S1198-743X(15)60017-9/pdf

- "Serious infections caused by Gram-positive pathogens are increasingly difficult to treat because of pathogens such as methicillin-resistant *Staphylococcus aureus* (MRSA), vancomycin-resistant enterococci (VRE) and penicillin-resistant *Streptococcus pneumonia*. The more recent emergence of vancomycin-intermediate and –resistant MRSA (VISA and VRSA) has further compromised treatment options."

Merrett, G. (2013). *Tackling antibiotic resistance for greater global health security.* Centre on Global Health Security. https://www.chathamhouse.org/sites/files/chathamhouse/public/Research/Global%20Health/1013bp_antibioticresistance.pdf

- "Integrated efforts involving academia, policy-makers, industry and interest groups will be required to produce a global political response with strong leadership, based on a coherent set of priorities and actions."
- In addition to the usual causes of ABR infections, this report also cites "Availability of poor quality antibiotics" and "Increased global travel, medical tourism and travel"
- "An important leverage point in working with the agricultural sector is engaging the food industry on this issue. So far [in the USA] this not been successful…and appears to be a highly politicized issue.

Mezzatesta, M., et al. (2012). Enterobacter cloacae complex: Clinical impact and emerging antibiotic resistance. *Future Mirobiology.* 7(7). pg. 887-902. http://www.ncbi.nlm.nih.gov/pubmed/22827309

- "Although the *E. cloacae* complex strains are among the most common *Enterobacter* spp. Causing nosocomial bloodstream infections in the last decade, little is known about their virulence-associated properties. By contrast, much has been published on the antibiotic-resistance features of these microorganisms."

- "Many other resistance determinants that are able to render ineffective almost all antibiotic families have been recently acquired."

Miao, X., Bishay, F., Chen, M. and Metcalfe, C. (2004). Occurrence of antimicrobials in the final effluents of wastewater treatment plants in Canada. *Environmental Science and Technology*. 38(13). pg. 3533-41. http://pubs.acs.org/doi/abs/10.1021/es030653q

Miller, K. P. (2015a). *Bacterial communication and its role as a target for nanoparticle-based antimicrobial therapy.* (Doctoral dissertation). http://scholarcommons.sc.edu/etd/3188/

Miller, K. P., Wang, L., Chen, Y-P., et al. (2015b). Engineering nanoparticles to silence bacterial communication. *Front. Microbiol.* 6(189). pg. 1-7. http://www.ncbi.nlm.nih.gov/pubmed/25806030

Mocan, L. (2013). Nanotechnology based platforms for the treatment of infectious diseases. *Biotechnology, Molecular Biology and Nanomedicine*. 1(2). pg. 25-30.

Mohney, Gillian. (September 21, 2016). UN leaders discuss dwindling options for antibiotic-resistant diseases. *ABC News*. http://abcnews.go.com/Health/leaders-discuss-dwindling-options-antibiotic-resistant-diseases/story?id=42252063

Montero, J. G., Lerma, F. A., Galleymore, P. R., et al. (2015). Combating resistance in intensive care: The multimodal approach of the Spanish ICU "Zero Resistance" program. *Critical Care*. 19(1). pg. 114. http://www.ncbi.nlm.nih.gov/pmc/articles/PMC4361202/

- "An ominous emerging threat is the appearance of Gram-negative microorganisms harboring new beta-lactamases that confer high-level resistance to all available classes of beta-lactam antibiotics."

Morens, D., Folkers, G. and Fauci, A. (2004). The challenge of emerging and re-emerging infectious diseases. *Nature*. 430. pg. 242-9. http://www.nature.com/nature/journal/v430/n6996/full/nature02759.html

- "About 15 million (>25%) of 57 million annual deaths worldwide are estimated to be related directly to infectious diseases."
- "The burden of morbidity (ill health) and mortality falls most heavily on people in developing countries, and particularly on infants and children (about three million children die each year from malaria and diarrhoeal diseases alone."

Morgenstern, M. Erichsen, C. Hackl, S., et al. (2016). Antibiotic resistance of commensal *Staphylococcus aureus* and coagulase-negative staphylococci in an international cohort of surgeons: A prospective point-prevalence study. *PLOS One*. 11(2). pg. 1-16. https://www.ncbi.nlm.nih.gov/pubmed/26840492

Moura, A., Henriques, I., Smalla, K. and Correia, A. (2010). Wastewater bacterial communities bring together broad-host range plasmids, integrons and a wide diversity of uncharacterized gene cassettes. *Research in Microbiology*. 161(1). pg. 58-66. http://www.ncbi.nlm.nih.gov/pubmed/20004718

- "Wastewater environments promote the development of bacterial communities that support and bring together different types of molecular elements that, in association, play a major role in bacterial adaptation and evolution."

Munir, M., Wong, K. and Xagoraraki, I. (2011). Release of antibiotic resistant bacteria and genes in the effluent and biosolids of five wastewater utilities in Michigan. *Water Research*. 45. pg. 681-93. http://www.ncbi.nlm.nih.gov/pubmed/20850863

- "Significant difference ($p<0.05$) was observed in concentration of ARGs (*tet*O and *Sul*I), and ARB in biosolids samples between the advanced treatment methods (anaerobic digestion and lime stabilization) and the conventional dewatering and gravity thickening methods. Daily release loads of ARGs and ARB in the environment were found to be higher through biosolids relative to effluents."

Nair, S. and Simidu, U. (1987). Distribution and significance of heterotrophic marine bacteria with antibacterial activity. *Applied and Environmental Microbiology*. 53(12). pg. 2957-62. http://www.ncbi.nlm.nih.gov/pubmed/3435149

- "Many marine heterotrophic bacteria are known to produce antibacterial substances which inhibit or kill other bacteria."
- "Isolation and characterization of antibiotic components have been carried out by various researchers."
- "Bacteria with antibacterial activity were isolated from seawater, sediments, phytoplankton, and zooplankton of Suruga, Sagami, and Tokyo Bays and from soft corals and sponges collected from the Taiwan coast. Of the 726 strains isolated, 37 showed antibacterial activity against either *Vibrio parahaemolyticus* (ATCC 17802) or *Staphylococcus aureus* (P209)."
- "Relatively high numbers of strains with antibacterial activity were associated with phytoplankton. Among the zooplankton isolates, cladocerans harbored the maximum number of antibacterial strains."

TABLE 1. Percentage of bacterial strains exhibiting antibacterial activity isolated from different sources

Source (n)	% (no.) of antibacterial strains		Total %	
	Antivi-brio	Antistaphylo-coccus	Antivi-brio	Antistaphylo-coccus
Water				
Free (126)	2.4	3.2	12.5	13.3
Attached (116)	6.0	6.9	29.1	26.7
Sediment (39)	2.7	0.0	4.2	0.0
Phytoplankton (40)	10.0	25.0	16.7	33.3
Zooplankton (262)	3.1	2.7	33.3	23.3
Sponges (143)	0.7	0.7	4.2	3.3
Total (726)	3.3 (24)	4.1 (30)	100	100

Nakada, N., Tanishima, T., Shinohara, H., Kiri, K.and Takada, H. (2006). Pharmaceutical chemicals and endocrine disrupters in municipal wastewater in Tokyo and their removal during activated sludge treatment. *Water Research*. 40(17). pg. 3297-303. http://www.ncbi.nlm.nih.gov/pubmed/16938339

- "We investigated the efficiencies of removal of 24 pharmaceutically active compounds (PhACs) during sand filtration and ozonation in an operating municipal sewage treatment plant (STP)."
- "The target compounds were 2 phenolic antiseptics (thymol, triclosan), 5 acidic analgesics or anti-inflammatories (ibuprofen, naproxen, ketoprofen, fenoprofen, mefenamic acid), 4 amide pharmaceuticals (propyphenazone, crotamiton, carbamazepine, diethyltouluamide), 7 antibiotics (sulfapyridine, sulfamethoxazole, trimethoprim, azithromycin, erythromycin anhydride, clarithromycin, roxithromycin), 3 phenolic endocrine-disrupting chemicals (EDCs) (nonylphenol:NP, octylphenol:OP, bisphenol A: BPA), and 3 natural estrogens (17 β-estradiol:E2, estrone:E1, estriol:E3)."
- "The combination of ozonation and sand filtration with activated sludge treatment gave efficient removal (>80%) of most of the target compounds."

Nandi, S., Maurer, J. J., Hofacre, C. and Summers, A. O. (2004). Gram-positive bacteria are a major reservoir of class 1 antibiotic resistance integrons in poultry litter. *Proceedings of the National Academy of Sciences*. 10(18). pg. 7118-22. www.pnas.org/cgi/doi/10.1073/pnas.0306466101

- "Formerly assumed barriers to intergenus exchange are far from absolute."
- "We...demonstrate the value of direct cultivation-independent quantification of target genes as a tool for the discovery of unexpected relationships in complex microbial ecosystems."

National Resources Defense Council. (2010). *Dosed without prescription: Preventing pharmaceutical contamination of our nation's drinking water*. NRDC. https://www.nrdc.org/health/files/dosed4pgr.pdf

- "Prescription drugs can enter water through manufacturing waste, human or animal excretion, runoff from animal feeding operations, leaching from municipal landfills, or improper disposal."
- "In March 2008 the Associated Press reported that pharmaceutical residues had been detected in the drinking water of 24 major metropolitan areas across the country serving 41 million people; detected drugs included antibiotics, anticonvulsants, and mood stabilizers."
- "Samples taken from 139 streams in 30 states in 1999-2000 by the U.S. Geologic Survey identified both organic wastewater contaminants and pharmaceuticals in 80 percent of the sampled sites. The range of drugs found in the water included antibiotics, hypertensive and cholesterol-lowering drugs, antidepressants, analgesics, steroids, caffeine, and reproductive hormones."
- "A large portion of the pharmaceuticals in our water come from the improper disposal of unused or unwanted drugs by households and medical facilities. Most people either fish them down the toilet or throw them in the trash."
- "One survey in Washington State found that over 65 percent of pharmaceutical waste was coming from 'specialty outpatient' facilities, more than 20 percent from hospitals, and about 5 percent coming from nursing homes, boarding homes, and retail pharmacies."

Nelson, D. J., Abutaleb, Y. and McNeill, R. (September 7, 2016). As if the killer got away. *Reuters*. http://www.reuters.com/investigates/special-report/usa-uncounted-surveillance/

Nordmann, P., Naas, T. and Poirel, L. (2011). Global spread of Carbapenemase-producing Enterobacteriaceae. *Emerging Infectious Diseases*. 17(10). pg. 1791-98. http://wwwnc.cdc.gov/eid/article/17/10/11-0655_article

- "*Enterobacteriaceae* are inhabitants of the intestinal flora and are among the most common human pathogens, causing infections such as cystitis and pyelonephritis with fever, septicemia, pneumonia, peritonitis, meningitis, and device-associated infections."
- "Modulation of the factors that enhance spread of carbapenemase producers in the community is difficult because these factors are multiple and are associated with lack of hygiene, overuse and over-the-counter use of antibacterial drugs, and increased worldwide travel…Many countries that are likely to be their main reservoirs have not established any search protocol for their detection."
- "The second epidemic will likely be caused mainly by nosocomial carbapenemasse producers in *K. pneumonia* of all types (KPC, IMP, VIM, NDM,

and OXA-48). It is likely that in certain countries high rates of different types of carapenemase producers may already exist, for example, in Greece (VIM and KPC) and in the Indian subcontinent (NDM, KPC, OXA-181)."

O'Fallon, E., Pop-Vicas, A. and D'Agata, E. (2009). The emerging threat of multidrug-resistant gram-negative organisms in long-term care facilities. *Journals of Gerontology Series: Biological Sciences and Medical Sciences.* 64A(1). pg. 138-41. http://www.ncbi.nlm.nih.gov/pmc/articles/PMC2691192/

- "The rapid and ongoing spread of antimicrobial-resistant bacteria throughout all health care institutions is considered a critical medical and public health issue. Residents of long-term care facilities (LTCF) are one of the main reservoirs of antimicrobial-resistant bacteria with reported prevalence rates similar to patients in the intensive care unit."
- "*Results.* A total of 1,661 clinical cultures were included in the analysis. MDRGN were recovered from 180 (10.8%) cultures, MRSA from 104 (6.3%), and VRE from 11 (0.6%) MDRGN were isolated more frequently than MRSA or VRE throughout the study period. The prevalence of MDRGN increased significantly from 7% in 2003 to 13% in 2005 throughout the study period. The prevalence of MDRGN increased significantly from 7% in 2003 to 13% in 2005 *(p = .001)*. More than 80% of MDRGN isolates were resistant to ciprofloxacin, TMP/SMX, and ampicillin/sulbactam. Resistance to three, four, and five or more antimicrobials were identified among 122 (67.8%), 47 (26.1%), and 11 (6.1%) MDRGN isolates, respectively."
- "*Conclusions.* Rates of MDRGN exceeded those of MRSA and VRE and increased throughout the study period. Resistance to multiple, commonly prescribed antimicrobials among MDRGN raises concerns about therapeutic options available to treat MDRGN infections among LTCF residents. The novel findings provided from this study emphasize the urgent need for further research on the epidemiology of MDRGN in the LTCF setting, including transmission patterns, the natural history of MDRGN colonization, rates of infection and associated morbidity and mortality."

O'Flaherty, S., Ross, R. P., Meaney, W. et. al (2005). Potential of the polyvalent anti-Staphylococcus bacteriophage K for control of antibiotic-resistant Staphylococci from hospitals. *Applied and Environmental Microbiology.* 71(4). pg. 1836-42. http://aem.asm.org/content/71/4/1836.full

- "The increasing prevalence of antibiotic-resistant staphylococci has prompted the need for antibacterial controls other than antibiotics."

- "Model in situ hand wash studies using a phage-enriched wash solution resulted in a 100-fold reduction in staphylococcal numbers on human skin by comparison with numbers remaining after washing in phage-free solution. Infusion of the phage into a nonimmunogenic bismuth-based cream resulted in strong anti-Staphylococcus activity from the cream on plates and in broth."

Okami, Y. (1984). Marine microorganisms as a source of bioactive substances. In: *Current perspectives in microbial ecology.* Klug, M. J. and Reddy, C. A. Eds. American Society for Microbiology. https://www.researchgate.net/publication/258429305_Marine_Microorganisms_as_a_source_of_bioactive_agents

Okeke, et al. (1999). Socioeconomic and behavioral factors leading to acquired bacterial resistance to antibiotics in developing countries. *Emerging Infectious Diseases.* 5(2). pg. 18-27.

- "Complex socioeconomic and behavioral factors [are] associated with antibiotic resistance, particularly regarding diarrheal and respiratory pathogens, in developing tropical countries."
- "Armed conflicts have recently led to a breakdown in health services and sanitation and rapid dissemination of resistant pathogens, particularly in sub-Saharan Africa and Asia."
- This article has an extensive bibliography.

Oshinsky, David M. (2005). *Polio: An American story.* Oxford University Press, Cambridge, MA.

Otter, J. and French, G. (2008). Survival of nosocomial bacteria and spores on surfaces and inactivation by hydrogen peroxide vapor. *Journal of Clinical Microbiology*, 47(1). pg. 205-7. http://www.ncbi.nlm.nih.gov/pmc/articles/PMC2620839/

- "With inocula of 6 to 7 log10 CFU, most vegetative bacteria and spores tested survived on surfaces for more than 5 weeks, but all were inactivated within 90 min of exposure to hydrogen peroxide vapor in a 100-m3 test room even in the presence of 0.3% bovine serum albumin to simulate biological soiling."

Pallecchi, L., Bartoloni, A., and Riccobono, E., et al. (2012). Quinolone resistance in absence of selective pressure: The experience of a very remote community in the Amazon forest. *PLOS Neglected Tropical Diseases.* 6(8). pg. 1-7. http://journals.plos.org/plosntds/article?id=10.1371/journal.pntd.0001790

- "Remoteness and absence of antibiotic selective pressure did not protect the community from the remarkable emergence of quinolone resistance in *E.*

coli…Improving sanitation and water/food safety are urgently needed…in resource–limited countries, as control strategies based only on antibiotic restriction policies are unlikely to succeed in those settings."

Pallecchi, L., Lucchetti, C., Bartoloni, A. et al. (2007). Population structure and resistance genes in antibiotic-resistant bacteria from a remote community with minimal antibiotic exposure . *Antimicrobial Agents and Chemotherapy.* 51(4). pg. 1179-84. http://www.ncbi.nlm.nih.gov/pmc/articles/PMC1855465/

- "The reasons for maintaining the high prevalence of resistance in the absence of antibiotic use remain unexplained…Strategies based only on antibiotic restriction policies are unlikely to fully succeed for these types of resistant strains and resistance genes."

Pang, B., Du, P., Zhou, Z., et al. (2016). The transmission and antibiotic resistance variation in a multiple drug resistance clade of *Vibrio cholera* circulating in multiple countries in Asia. *PLOS One.* pg. 3-11. http://journals.plos.org/plosone/article?id=10.1371/journal.pone.0149742

Pathak, S. and Gopal, K. (2008). Prevalence of bacterial contamination with antibiotic-resistant and enterotoxigenic fecal coliforms in treated drinking water. *Journal of Toxicology and Environmental Health.* 71. pg. 427-33. http://www.ncbi.nlm.nih.gov/pubmed/18306089

Patterson, D. L. (2006). Resistance in gram-negative bacteria: Enterobacteriaceae. *American Journal of Infection Control.* 34(5). pg. S20-8.

- "Carbapenem resistance, although rare, appears to be increasing. Particularly troublesome is the emergence of KPC-type carbapenemases in New York City. Better antibiotic stewardship and infection control are needed to prevent further spread of ESBLs and other forms of resistance in Enterobacteriaceae throughout the world."

Pei, R., Kim, S., Carlson, K., et al. (2006). Effect of river landscape on the sediment concentrations of antibiotics and corresponding antibiotic resistance genes (ARG). *Water Research.* 40. pg. 2427-35. http://www.engr.colostate.edu/~apruden/resume/Pei%20et%20al%20Water%20Researc h%202006.pdf

Pei, R., Cha, J., Carlson, K., et al. (2007). Response of antibiotic resistance genes (ARG) to biological treatment in dairy lagoon water. *Environmental Science and Technology.* 41. pg. 5108-13. http://www.ncbi.nlm.nih.gov/pubmed/17711231

Percival, S. L., Bowler, P. G. and Russell, D. (2005). Bacterial resistance to silver in wound care. *Journal of Hospital Infection*. 60. pg. 1-7. http://www.ncbi.nlm.nih.gov/pubmed/15823649

- "Concerns associated with the overuse of silver and the consequent emergence of bacterial resistance are being raised...[including] the likelihood of widespread resistance to silver and the potential for silver to induce cross-resistance to antibiotics."

Perez, F., Hujer, A. M., Hujer, K. M., et al. (2007). Global challenge of multidrug-resistant acinetobacter baumannii. *Antimicrobial Agents and Chemotherapy*. 51(10). pg. 3471-84. http://aac.asm.org/content/51/10/3471.full

- "We may soon be facing the end of the 'antibiotic era.' The initial and seemingly unstoppable success of antibiotics, the fruit of human ingenuity, has been countered by...the emergence of many genera of bacteria that are resistant to all antibiotics. The genus *Acinetobacter* epitomizes this trend and deserves close attention."
- "There are reports of MDR *A. baumannii* from hospitals in Europe, North America, Argentina, Brazil, China, Taiwan, Hong Kong, Japan, and Korea and from areas as remote as Tahiti in the South Pacific."
- "More recently, cases of United Kingdom and U.S. military and nonmilitary personnel returning from operations in Iraq and Afghanistan and harboring infections caused by MDR *A. baumannii* are receiving increased attention."

Perni, S., Piccirillo, C., Pratten, J., et al. (2009). The antimicrobial properties of light-activated polymers containing methylene blue and gold nanoparticles. *Biomaterials*. 30(1). pg. 89-93. http://www.sciencedirect.com/science/article/pii/S0142961208006807

Petrovic, M., Lopez de Alda, M. J., Diaz-Cruz, S., et al. (2009). Fate and removal of pharmaceuticals and illicit drugs in conventional and membrane bioreactor wastewater treatment plants and by riverbank filtration. *Philosophical Transactions Of The Royal Society*. 367. pg. 3979-4003. http://rsta.royalsocietypublishing.org/content/367/1904/3979

- "Pharmaceutically active compounds (PhACs) and drugs of abuse (Das) are two important groups of emerging environmental contaminants that have raised an increasing interest in the scientific community."
- "Some compounds are not efficiently removed during wastewater treatment processes, being able to reach surface and groundwater and subsequently, drinking waters."

78

Pfaller, M. A. and Diekema, D. J. (2004). Rare and emerging opportunistic fungal pathogens: concern for resistance beyond *Candida albicans* and *Aspergillus fumigatus*. *Journal of Clinical Microbiology*. 42(10). pg. 4419-31. http://jcm.asm.org/content/42/10/4419.full

- "The frequency of invasive mycoses due to opportunistic fungal pathogens has increased significantly over the past two decades...Serious life-threatening infections are being reported with an ever increasing array of pathogens, including the well-known opportunists *Candida albicans, Cryptococcus neoformans,* and *Aspergillus fumigatus.*"

Podolsky, S. H. (2014). *The antibiotic era; reform, resistance, and the pursuit of a rational therapeutic.* Johns Hopkins University Press, Baltimore, MD.

Pollack, A. (February 27, 2010). Rising threat of infections unfazed by antibiotics. *The New York Times.* pg. B-1. http://www.nytimes.com/2010/02/27/business/27germ.html?_r=0

- "The bacteria [*Acinetobacter*] classified as Gram-negative because of their reaction to the so-called gram stain test, can cause severe pneumonia and infections of the urinary tract, bloodstream and other parts of the body. Their cell structure makes them more difficult to attack with antibiotics than gram-positive organisms like MRSA."
- "Meanwhile, New York City hospitals, perhaps because of the large number of patients they treat, have become the global breeding ground for another drug-resistant gram-negative germ, *Klebsiella pneumoniae.*"
- "MRSA remains the single most common source of hospital infections...it can also infect people outside the hospital."
- "By comparison, the drug-resistant gram-negative germs for the most part threaten only hospitalized patients whose immune systems are weak. The germs can survive for a long time on surfaces in the hospital and enter the body through wounds, catheters and ventilators."

Projan, S. J. (2003). Why is Pharma getting out of antibacterial drug discovery? *Current Opinion in Microbiology*. 6. pg. 427-30. http://www.ncbi.nlm.nih.gov/pubmed/14572532

Pruden, A., Pei, R., Storteboom, H. and Carlson, K. (2006). Antibiotic resistance genes as emerging contaminants: Studies in northern Colorado. *Environmental Science and Technology*. 40. pg. 7445-50. http://pubs.acs.org/doi/abs/10.1021/es0604131

- This study explores antibiotic resistance genes (ARGs).

- "In various environmental compartments in northern Colorado, including Cache La Poudre (Poudre) River sediments, irrigation ditches, dairy lagoons, and the effluents of wastewater recycling and drinking water treatment plant."
- "The following trend was observed with respect to ARG concentrations: dairy lagoon water > irrigation ditch water > urban/agriculturally impacted river sediments."

Quednau, M., et al. (1998). Antibiotic-resistant strains of *Enterococcus* isolated from Swedish and Danish retailed chicken and pork. *The Society for Applied Microbiology.* 84(6). pg. 1163-70. http://www.ncbi.nlm.nih.gov/pubmed/9717303

- "Seventy-three per cent of the *Enterococcus* isolates from Swedish chicken were resistant to one or more of the tested antibiotics."
- "For *Ent. Faecium*, the situation was even worse; all were resistant to chloramphenicol and high resistance (50-90% of the isolates) was found to penicillin V, ampicillin, tetracycline, erythromycin, norfloxacin and trimethoprim."
- "All of the vancomycin-resistant isolates found, except one, were also resistant to erythromycin."

Rahimi, E., Momtaz, H., Sharifzadeh, A., et al. (2012). Prevalence and antimicrobial resistance of *Listeria* species isolated from traditional dairy products in Chahar Mahal & Bakhtiy Ari, Iran. *Bulgarian Journal of Veterinary Medicine.* 15(2). pg. 115-22.

- "The results provide information about the contamination levels of traditional dairy products in one of the provinces of Iran and highlight the emergence of multi-drug resistant *Listeria* in the environment."

Rai, V. R. and Bai, A. J. (2011). Nanoparticles and their potential application as antimicrobials. In: *Science against microbial pathogens: Communicating Current research and technological advances*. Formatex Research Center, Badajoz, Spain. http://citeseerx.ist.psu.edu/viewdoc/download?doi=10.1.1.459.8922&rep=rep1&type=pdf

- "Nanoparticles have unique and well defined physical and chemical properties which can be manipulated suitably for desired applications."
- "The application of nanoparticles as antimicrobials is gaining relevance in prophylaxis and therapeutics, in medical devices, food industry and textile fabrics. The problems related to toxicity of nanoparticles will be addressed in brief."
- Use of the term "synthetic nanoparticles" would be helpful.

- "Studies conducted on the NP-induced toxicity have revealed that the metal-based nanoparticles can affect the biological behavior at the organ, tissue, cellular, subcellular, and protein levels.
- Metal synthetic nanoparticles discussed include…silver, gold, magnesium oxide, copper oxide, aluminum, titanium dioxide and zinc oxide.

Ranghar, S., Sirohi, P., Verma, P. and Agarwal, V. (2014). Nanoparticle-based drug delivery systems: Promising approaches against infections. *Brazilian Archives of Biology and Technology*. 57(2). pg. 209-22.

- "The use of conventional antimicrobial agents…to combat infectious diseases…[is] associated with problems such as the development of multiple drug resistance and adverse side effects…The inefficient traditional drug delivery system results in inadequate therapeutic index, low bioavailability of drugs and many other limitations."
- "In this regard, antimicrobial nanoparticles and nanosized drug delivery carriers have emerged as potent effective agents against infections… [including] nanoparticle systems for antimicrobial drug delivery and use of these systems for antimicrobial drug delivery and use of these systems for delivery of various antimicrobial agents."
- Antimicrobial nanoparticles – the hope of the future to counteract antibiotic winter.

Reardon, S. (2014). Antibiotic resistance sweeping developing world. *Nature*. 509. pg. 141-2. http://www.nature.com/news/antibiotic-resistance-sweeping-developing-world-1.15171

- "Around the globe, overuse of drugs has created resistant strains of deadly bacteria – and they could be a greater threat in poorer nations than in richer ones, owing in part to a lack of regulation."
- "The problem also seems to be particularly acute in the emerging economies known as the 'BRIC' states: Brazil, Russia, India and China, says Keith Klugman, an epidemiologist for the Bill and Melinda Gates Foundation in Seattle, Washington."
- "Researchers do not know what factors have caused resistance to grow so rapidly in developing nations. For instance, it is not clear to what extent the rise of resistance has been spurred by the use of antibiotics for growth promotion in livestock, or by the release of antibiotics into wastewater by drug-manufacturers in countries such as India."

Reinert, R., Low, D., Rossi, F., et al. (2007). Antimicrobial susceptibility among organisms from the Asia/Pacific Rim, Europe and Latin and North America collected as part of TEST and the in vitro activity of tigecycline. *Journal of Antimicrobial Chemotherapy.* 60(5). pg. 1018-29. http://jac.oxfordjournals.org/content/60/5/1018.long

- "Widespread inappropriate use of antimicrobial agents in the hospital setting has resulted in the emergence of resistance in nosocomial organisms, and lack of adherence to hygiene practices has facilitated their dissemination."
- "The key to antimicrobial development has been to design agents that elude the main bacterial resistance mechanisms. One such agent is tigecycline, a tetracycline analogue in the new antimicrobial class of glycyclines."
- "The Tigecycline Evaluation and Surveillance Trial (TEST) is a global multicenter study designed to compare the *in vitro* activity of tigecycline with established antimicrobial agents against a range of clinically important organisms."
- "Surveillance of antimicrobial resistance is essential to understand trends in resistance so as to develop judicious treatment guidelines and to assess the effectiveness of interventions. There are a number of international surveillance studies currently in operation, perhaps the most widely known being The Surveillance Network (TSN) and SENTRY. TEST covers a large geographic area, involves a wide range of Gram-positive and Gram-negative organisms and with 3 years of operation currently contains more than 35,000 isolations in its database."
- "A comprehensive worldwide survey of anti-microbial susceptibility in so far as data was available between January and August 2006."
- The study was funded by Wyeth Pharmaceuticals.

Rice, L. (2006). Antimicrobial resistance in gram-positive bacteria. *The American Journal of Medicine.* 119(6A). pg. S11-9. http://www.ncbi.nlm.nih.gov/pubmed/16735146

- "In the United States, approximately 60% of staphylococcal infections in the intensive care unit are now caused by MRSA, and percentages continue to rise. Outbreaks of hospital-acquired MRSA (HA-MRSA) are typically the result of clonal spread by MRSA being transferred from patient to patient, frequently using healthcare personnel as intermediaries. HA-MRSA strains are generally multidrug resistant…The mechanisms of methicillin resistance are the same for CA-MRSA and HA-MRSA."

Riesenfeld, C., Goodman, R., and Handelsman, J. (2004). Uncultured soil bacteria are a reservoir of new antibiotic resistance genes. *Environmental Microbiology*. 6(9). Pg. 981-989. http://www.ncbi.nlm.nih.gov/pubmed/15305923

- "Antibiotic resistance genes are typically isolated by cloning from cultured bacteria or by polymerase chain reaction (PCR) amplification from environmental samples."
- "Based on the predicted amino acid sequences of the resistance genes the resistance mechanisms include efflux of tetracycline and inactivation of aminoglycoside antibiotics by phosphorylation and acetylation."
- "The results indicate that soil bacteria are a reservoir of antibiotic resistance genes with greater genetic diversity than previously accounted for."

Rizzo, L., Manaia, C., Merlin, C. et al. (2013). Urban wastewater treatment plants as hotspots for antibiotic resistant bacteria and genes spread into the environment: a review. *Science of the Total Environment*. 447. pg. 345-60. http://www.sciencedirect.com/science/article/pii/S0048969713000429

- "Urban wastewater treatment plants (UWTPs) are among the main sources of antibiotics' release into the environment. The occurrence of antibiotics may promote the selection of antibiotic resistance genes (ARGs) and antibiotic resistant bacteria(ARB)."
- "The mechanisms by which biological processes influence the development/selection of ARB and ARGs transfer are still poorly understood."
- "Some studies showed that conventional UWTPs may positively affect ARB spread and selection as well as ARG transfer."
- "Demonstrating ARG transfer in complex environments remains a difficult task although indispensable for an adequate risk assessment of resistance spread in UWTPs."
- "All known types of antibiotic resistance mechanisms are represented in UWTP, suggesting the relevance of these facilities as reservoirs and environmental suppliers of genetic determinants of resistance."

Rosenfeld, W. and ZoBell, C. (1947). Antibiotic production by marine organisms. *Journal of Bacteriology*. 54. pg. 393-8. http://www.ncbi.nlm.nih.gov/pmc/articles/PMC526565/

Rysz, M. and Alvarez, P. (2004). Amplification and attenuation of tetracycline resistance in soil bacteria: Aquifer column experiments. *Water Research*. 38. pg. 3705-12. http://alvarez.rice.edu/files/2012/02/56.pdf

Salyers, A. A., Gupta, A. and Wang, Y. (2004). Human intestinal bacteria as reservoirs for antibiotic resistance genes. *Trends in Microbiology*. 12. pg. 412-6.
http://www.congrex.ch/2006/escmidschool2006/pdf/edu_mat_2006_13.pdf

Salyers, A. A. and Whitt, D. D. (2005). Revenge of the microbes: How bacterial resistance is undermining the antibiotic miracle. *Emerging Infectious Diseases*. 11(10).

- "Provides the scientific information readers will need to form opinions and make informed decisions regarding the use of antibiotics. Examines specific antibiotics and controversies in a real-life context; presents accounts of positions on all sides of the public policy debate; and discusses less common issues such as what happens to antibiotics once they are released into the environment."

Sapkota, A., Lefferts, L., McKenzie, S., et al. (2007). What do we feed to food-production animals? A review of animal feed ingredients and their potential impacts on human health. *Environmental Health Perspectives*. 115. pg. 663-70.
http://www.ncbi.nlm.nih.gov/pmc/articles/PMC1867957/

Sapkota, A., et al. (2011). Lower prevalence of antibiotic-resistant Enterococci on U.S. conventional poultry farms that transitioned to organic processes. *Environmental Health Perspectives*. 119(11). pg. 1622-8.
http://www.ncbi.nlm.nih.gov/pmc/articles/PMC3226496/

- "The voluntary removal of antibiotics from large-scale U.S. poultry farms that transition to organic practices is associated with a lower prevalence of antibiotic-resistant and MDR Enterococcus."
- "Organic certification standards need to be met before the first day of life. Thus, some breeder facilities that supply eggs to hatcheries, and hatcheries that ultimately produce "organic" chicks, do not have to meet any organic standards and can therefore use antibiotics among breeder stocks and inject antibiotics into eggs. These practices can result in exposures to antibiotics among "organic" broilers before the first day of life."
- "Organic broilers can be exposed to antibiotic-resistant bacteria through feed and water. In U.S. conventional poultry production, antibiotics are administered for therapeutic, prophylactic, and non-therapeutic purposes…The use of antimicrobials in conventional U.S. poultry production (on a per bird basis) increased by 307% from 1985 to the late 1990's, with the use of nontherapeutic antimicrobial growth promoters (AGPs) accounting for a significant portion of this use (Mellon et al. 2001)."

Sarmah, A., Myer, M. and Boxall, A. (2006). A global perspective on the use, sales, exposure pathways, occurrence, fate and effects of veterinary antibiotics (VAs) in the

environment. *Chemosphere*. 65. pg. 725-59.
http://www.ncbi.nlm.nih.gov/pubmed/16677683

Schulter, A., Szczepanowski, R. and Puhler, A. (2007). Genomics of IncP-1 antibiotic resistance plasmids isolated from wastewater treatment plants provides evidence for a widely accessible drug resistance gene pool. *FEMS Microbiology Review*. 31. pg. 449-77. http://onlinelibrary.wiley.com/doi/10.1111/j.1574-6976.2007.00074.x/epdf

Schmidt, A., Bruun, M., Dalsgaard, I. and Larsen, J. (2001). Incidence, distribution, and spread of tetracycline resistance determinants and integrin-associated antibiotic resistance genes among motile aeromonads from a fish farming environment. *Applied Environmental Microbiology*. 67. pg. 5675-82.
http://www.ncbi.nlm.nih.gov/pmc/articles/PMC93359/

Schwartz, T., Kohnen, W., Jansen, B. and Obst, U. (2003). Detection of antibiotic-resistant bacteria and their resistance genes in wastewater, surface water, and drinking water biofilms. *FEMS Microbiology and Ecology*. 43. pg. 325-35.
http://onlinelibrary.wiley.com/doi/10.1111/j.1574-6941.2003.tb01073.x/pdf

Scientific Committee on Consumer Safety (SCCS). (22 June 2010). *Opinion on triclosan (antimicrobial resistance)*.
http://ec.europa.eu/health/scientific_committees/consumer_safety/docs/sccs_o_023.pdf

- A definitive survey of the production, use, and fate of triclosan and the mechanisms of bacterial resistance to triclosan.
- "Several distinct hazards have been identified: (i) the effect of triclosan on the triggering/regulation of resistance genes in bacteria (ii) the existence of defined mechanisms that can promote resistance and cross-resistance to biocides and antibiotics in bacteria."
- "It is not possible to quantify the risk associated with triclosan (including its use in cosmetics) in terms of development of antimicrobial resistance."
- This publication contains a comprehensive bibliography on the uses, effects, and possible impact of triclosan.

Shah, Sonia. (2016). *Pandemic: Tracking contagions, from cholera to ebola and beyond*. Sarah Crichton Books, NY.

Shallcross, Laura. (2014). Antibiotic overuse: A key driver of antimicrobial resistance. *British Journal of General Practice*. 64(629). pg. 604-5.
http://www.ncbi.nlm.nih.gov/pmc/articles/PMC4240113/

- "The problems of antimicrobial resistance will only be solved through global cooperation and mutual support from governments across the world working through the relevant United Nations organizations, the World Health Organization, the Food and Agriculture Organization, and the inter-governmental World Organization for Animal Health (OIE)."

Shelton, C. D. (2014). *Antibiotics: A limited resource*. Choice Publishing House, Drogheda, Ireland.

- "We are becoming increasingly more vulnerable to the indiscriminate use of antibiotics, from antibiotics used in the food industry to 'beef' up our animals, to people taking antibiotics for minor health issues."

Shiba, T. and Taga, N. (1980). Heterotrophic bacteria attached to seaweeds. *Journal of Experimental Marine Biology and Ecology*. 47. pg. 251-8. http://www.sciencedirect.com/science/article/pii/0022098180900428

Shenold, C. (2014). *Bacterial resistance: are we running out of antibiotics?* CME Resource/NetCE, Sacramento, CA.

- "The problem of multidrug-resistant microbial infection remains a ubiquitous and complex issue for communities and hospitals. Each decade seems to usher in a new generation of common bacterial pathogens that have become resistant to available antibiotics."

Siegel, R. (2008). Emerging gram-negative antibiotic resistance: Daunting challenges, declining sensitivities, and dire consequences. *Respiratory Care*. 53(4). http://www.ncbi.nlm.nih.gov/pubmed/18364060

- "Emerging antibiotic resistance has created a major public health dilemma, compounded by a dearth of new antibiotic options. Multidrug-resistant Gram-negative organisms have received less attention than Gram-positive threats, such as methicillin-resistant *Staphylococcus aureus*, but are just as menacing…Carbapenems, currently the most successful class of antibiotics, are showing signs of vulnerability."

Sieradzki, K., et al. (1999). The development of Vancomycin resistance in a patient with methicillin-resistant Staphylococcus Aureus infection. *Massachusetts Medical Society*. 340(7). http://www.nejm.org/doi/full/10.1056/NEJM199902183400704

- "Over the past two decades, vancomycin has been considered the antibiotic of choice for methicillin-resistant *Staphylococcus aureus* (MRSA) infections."
- "Recent reports describing the therapeutic failure of vancomycin for MRSA infections have aroused considerable concern regarding the emergence of MRSA strains for which there will be no effective therapy."

"The mechanism of reduced susceptibility in these staphylococcal strains has not been identified, although data indicate that it is not the same as the vancomycin-resistance mechanism in enterococcal strains."

Sieradzki, K., et al. (1999). The development of vancomycin resistance in a patient with methicillin-resistant staphylococcus aureus infection. *New England Journal of Medicine.* 340. Pg. 517-523. http://www.nejm.org/doi/full/10.1056/NEJM199902183400704

- "Over the past two decades, vancomycin has been considered the antibiotic of choice for methicillin-resistant *Staphylococcus aureus* (MRSA) infections."
- "Recent reports describing the therapeutic failure of vancomycin for MRSA infections have aroused considerable concern regarding the emergence of MRSA strains for which there will be no effective therapy."
- "The mechanism of reduced susceptibility in these staphylococcal strains has not been identified, although data indicate that it is not the same as the vancomycin-resistance mechanism in enterococcal strains."

Singh, H., Arora, E., Thangaraju, P., et al. (2013). Antimicrobial resistance: New patterns, emerging concepts and prevention. *Journal of Rational Pharmacotherapeutics Research* . 1(2). pg. 95-99. http://isrpt.co.in/archives/vol1_no2/4-Rational%20Pharmacotherapeutics.pdf

- "Antimicrobial resistance is the ability of a microorganism to survive and reproduce in the presence of antibiotic doses that were previously thought effective against them. It is defined as bacteria that are not inhibited by usually achievable systemic concentration of an agent with normal dosage schedule and/or fall in the minimum inhibitory concentration ranges. Multiple drug-resistance is defined as the resistance to two or more drugs or drug classes. Acquisition of resistance to one antibiotic conferring resistance to another antibiotic, to which the organism has not been exposed, is called cross resistance."

Skold, O. (2011). *Antibiotics and antibiotic resistance.* Wiley Publishing, Hoboken, NJ.

Sosa, A., Byarugaba, D. K., Ama´bile-Cuevas, A., et al., eds. (2010). *Antimicrobial resistance in developing countries.* Springer Science & Business Media, Berlin, Germany.

- This 539 page text is a comprehensive review of anti-microbial resistance as it "relates to the developing countries" in Asia, Africa and Latin America.

- The subject groups and its 30 chapters are: "General Issues in Antimicrobial Resistance, The Human Impact of Resistance, Antimicrobial Use and Misuse, Cost, Policy, and Regulation of Antimicrobials [and] Strategies to Contain Antimicrobial Resistance."

Spellberg, B., et al. (2007). Societal costs versus savings from wild-card patent extension legislation to spur critically needed antibiotic development. *Infection*. 35(3). pg. 167-74. http://www.ncbi.nlm.nih.gov/pubmed/17565458

- "[Based on the extension of] the patient…The Infectious Diseases Society of America (IDSA) has released a white paper that proposes incentives to stimulate critically needed antibiotic development by pharmaceutical companies….by a 'wild-card patent extension' program…the patent on a drug within their active portfolio."
- "We conservatively estimate that wild-card patent extension applied to one new antibiotic would cost $7.7 billion over the first 2 years, and $3.9 billion over the next 18 years."

Spellberg, B., Guidos, R., Gilbert, D., et al. (2008). The epidemic of antibiotic-resistant infections: a call to action for the medical community from the Infectious Diseases Society of America. *Clinical Infectious Diseases*. 46(2). pg. 155-164. http://cid.oxfordjournals.org/content/46/2/155.full.pdf+html

- "Despite intensive public relations and lobbying efforts, it remains unclear whether sufficiently robust legislation will be enacted. In the meantime, microbes continue to become more resistant, the antibiotic pipeline continues to diminish, and the majority of the public remains unaware of this critical situation."
- "The result of insufficient federal funding; insufficient surveillance, prevention, and control; insufficient research and development activities; misguided regulation of antibiotics in agriculture and, in particular, for food animals; and insufficient overall coordination of US (and international) efforts could mean a literal return to the preantibiotic era for many types of infections. If we are to address the antimicrobial resistance crisis, a concerted, grassroots effort led by the medical community will be required."

Spellberg, B. (2009). *The global threat from deadly bacteria and our dwindling arsenal to fight them.* Prometheus Books, Amherst, NY.

Srinivasan, V., Nam, H., Nguyen, L., Tamilselvam, B., Murinda, S. and Oliver, S. (2005). Prevalence of antimicrobial resistance genes in *Listeria monocytogenes* isolated from dairy farms. *Foodborne Pathogens and Disease*. 2. pg. 201-11.

https://www.researchgate.net/publication/7605619_Prevalence_of_Antimicrobial_Resistance_Genes_in_Listeria_monocytogenes_Isolated_from_Dairy_Farms

Stewart, P., Costerton, J. (2001). Antibiotic resistance of bacteria in biofilms. *The Lancet*. 358. pg. 135-38. http://www.thelancet.com/pdfs/journals/lancet/PIIS0140-6736(01)05321-1.pdf

- "Bacteria that adhere to implanted medical devices or damaged tissue can encase themselves in a hydrated matrix of polysaccharide and protein, and form a slimy layer known as a biofilm. Antibiotic resistance of bacteria in the biofilm mode of growth contributes to the chronicity of infections such as those associated with implanted medical devices. The mechanisms of resistance in biofilms are different from the now familiar plasmids, transposons, and mutations that confer innate resistance to individual bacterial cells. In biofilms, resistance seems to depend on multicellular strategies."

Su, T-H. and Chen, P-J. (2012). Emerging hepatitis B virus infection in vaccinated populations: a rising concern. *Emerging Microbes and Infections*. 1(e27). pg. 1-4. http://www.nature.com/emi/journal/v1/n9/pdf/emi201228a.pdf

- "Hepatitis B virus (HBV) infection is the major cause of viral hepatitis and affects more than 350 million individuals worldwide."
- "Perinatal transmission is the major route of hepatitis B transmission in Asia, where the infection is endemic."

Suller, A. and Russell, A. (2000). Triclosan and antibiotic resistance in *Staphylococcus aureus*. *Journal of Antimicrobial Chemotherapy*. 46. pg. 11-8. http://jac.oxfordjournals.org/content/46/1/11.full.pdf+html

- "Triclosan (2,4,4 -trichloro-2 -hydroxydiphenyl ether) is an antimicrobial agent used in hygiene products, plastics and kitchenware, and for treating methicillin-resistant *Staphylococcus aureus* (MRSA) outbreaks. *S. aureus* strains with low-level resistance to triclosan have emerged. It has been claimed that strains with decreased susceptibility to biocides may also be less susceptible to antibiotics. We tested the susceptibility of *S. aureus* clinical isolates to triclosan and several antibiotics. Triclosan MICs ranged between 0.025 and 1 mg/L. Some, but not all, strains were resistant to several antibiotics and showed low-level triclosan resistance. *S. aureus* mutants with enhanced resistance to triclosan (1 mg/L) were isolated. In several cases this resistance was stably inherited in the absence of triclosan. These mutants were not more resistant than the parent strain to several antibiotics. Changes in triclosan MICs associated with the acquisition of a plasmid encoding mupirocin resistance were not observed, suggesting that the triclosan/mupirocin co-resistance seen in a previous study was not the result of a single resistance gene or separate genes on the same plasmid. The continuous exposure of a triclosan-sensitive S. aureus strain to sub-MIC concentrations of triclosan for 1 month did not result in decreased susceptibility to triclosan or to several antibiotics tested. Triclosan- induced potassium leakage and bactericidal effects on a triclosan-sensitive strain, a resistant strain and a strain selected for increased resistance were compared with those of non-growing organisms, exponentially growing organisms and organisms in the stationary phase. No significant differences between the strains were observed under these conditions despite their different MICs. Biocides have multiple target sites and so MICs often do not correlate with bactericidal activities. The ability of *S. aureus* to develop resistance to triclosan and the current view that triclosan may have a specific target in Escherichia coli, namely enoyl reductase, underline the need for more research on the mechanisms of action and resistance."

Szcepanowski, R., Krahn, I., Linke, B., et al. (2004). Antibiotic multiresistance plasmid pRSB101 isolated from a wastewater treatment plant is related to plasmids residing in phytopathogenic bacteria and carries eight different resistance determinants including a multidrug transport system. *Microbiology*. 150(11). pg. 3613-30. http://www.ncbi.nlm.nih.gov/pubmed/15528650

Szcepanowskic, R., Braun, S., Riedel, V., et al. (2005). The 120 592 bp IncG plsdmif pTDN107 isolated from a sewage-treatment plant encodes nine different antibiotic-resistance determinants, two iron-acquisition systems and other putative virulence-associated functions. *Microbiology*. 151. pg. 1095-111. http://www.ncbi.nlm.nih.gov/pubmed/15817778

Szewzyk, U., Szewyk, R. and Manz, W. (2000). Microbiological safety of drinking water. *Annual Review of Microbiology*. 54. pg. 81-127. http://www.annualreviews.org/doi/abs/10.1146/annurev.micro.54.1.81?journalCode=micro

Tavernise, S. and Grady, D. (May 27, 2016). An infection raises the specter of superbugs resistant to all antibiotics. *The New York Times*. http://www.nytimes.com/2016/05/27/health/infection-raises-specter-of-superbugs-resistant-to-all-antibiotics.html?_r=0

- "The bacteria are resistant to a drug called colistin, an old antibiotic that in the United States is held in reserve to treat especially dangerous infections that are resistant to a class of drugs called carbapenems. If carbapenem-resistant bacteria, called CRE, also pick up resistance to colistin, they will be unstoppable."

Tenover, F. (2001). Development and spread of bacterial resistance to antimicrobial agents: An overview. *Clinical Infectious Diseases*. 33(3). pg. S108-S115.

- "Twenty years ago, bacteria that were resistant to antimicrobial agents were easy to detect in the laboratory because the concentration of drug required to inhibit their growth was usually quite high and distinctly different from that of susceptible strains."
- "Emerging resistance has required adaptations and modifications of laboratory diagnostic techniques, empiric anti-infective therapy for such diseases as bacterial meningitis, and infection control measures in health care facilities of all kinds. Judicious use is imperative if we are to preserve our arsenal of antimicrobial agents into the next decade."
- "As of 2016, our arsenal of antimicrobial agents, with one possible exception no longer exists."

Teuber, M. (2001). Veterinary use and antibiotic-resistance. *Current Opinion in Microbiology*. 4. pg. 493-9. http://www.ncbi.nlm.nih.gov/pubmed/11587923

- "Globally, an estimated 50% of all antimicrobials serve veterinary purposes. Bacteria that inevitably develop antibiotic resistance in animals comprise food-borne pathogens, opportunistic pathogens and commensal bacteria. The same antibiotic resistance genes and gene transfer mechanisms can be found in the microfloras of animals and humans. Direct contact, food and water link animal and human habitats."

Tieyu, W., Yonglong, L, Hong, Z. and Yajuan, S. (2005). Contamination of persistent organic pollutants (POPs) and relevant management in China. *Environment International*. 31. pg. 813-21.

- "Low POP levels might be increased by biomagnification through the transmission process in the food chain. They can be easily accumulated in the organism to levels that can potentially injure human health as well as the environment."

Travis, J. (1994). Reviving the antibiotic miracle? *Science*. (264). pg. 360-62. http://www.ncbi.nlm.nih.gov/pubmed/8153615

Turos, E., Reddy, G., Greenhalgh, K., et al. (2007a). Penicillin-bound polyacrylate nanoparticles: Restoring the activity of ß-lactam antibiotics against MRSA. *Bioorganic & Medicinal Chemistry Letters*. 17. pg. 3468-72. http://www.freepaperdownload.us/1748/Article3547978.htm

Turos, E., Shim, J-Y., Wang, Y., et al. (2007b). Antibiotic-conjugated polyacrylate nanoparticles: New opportunities for development of anti-MRSA agents. *Bioorganic & Medicinal Chemistry Letters*. 17. pg. 53-6. http://biology.usf.edu/cmmb/abl/data/Turos%20Lim%202007%20BMCL.pdf

Tzialla, C., et al. (2015). Antimicrobial therapy in neonatal intensive care unit. *Italian Journal of Pediatrics*. 41(27). http://ijponline.biomedcentral.com/articles/10.1186/s13052-015-0117-7

- Severe infections represent the main cause of neonatal mortality accounting for more than one million neonatal deaths worldwide every year.
- "The benefits of antibiotic therapy when indicated are clearly enormous, but the continued use of antibiotics without any microbiological justification is dangerous and only leads to adverse events."
- "Of 6,956 very low birth weight (VLBW) infants (showing that) 56% of all infants received at least one course of antibiotic treatment, proven sepsis was diagnosed in only 21% of all infants."

Udikovic-Kolic, N., Wichmann, F., Broderick, N. A. and Handelsman, J. (2014). Bloom of resident antibiotic-resistant bacteria in soil following manure fertilization. *Proceedings of the National Academy of Sciences*. 111(42). pg. 15202-07. http://www.pnas.org/content/111/42/15202.abstract

- "The increasing prevalence of antibiotic-resistant bacteria is one of the most serious threats to public health in the 21st century…In this study, we found that dairy cow manure amendment enhanced the proliferation of resident antibiotic-resistant bacteria and genes encoding β-lactamases in soil even though the cows from which the manure was derived had not been treated with antibiotics."
- "Animal manure is an important reservoir of antibiotic-resistant bacteria, antibiotic-resistance genes (collectively known as the 'resistome'), and pathogens (2, 7-12)."
- "Antibiotic-resistant bacteria are also abundant in manure from animals with no history of antibiotic treatment, indicating the natural presence of bacteria intrinsically resistant to antibiotics in animal gastrointestinal tracts."

Unemo, Magnus and Nicholas, Robert. (2014). Emergence of multidrug-resistant, extensively drug-resistant and untreatable gonorrhea. *Future Microbiology*. 7(12). pg. 1401. http://www.futuremedicine.com/doi/abs/10.2217/fmb.12.117

- "The new superbug Neisseria gonorrhoeae has retained resistance to antimicrobials previously recommended for first-line treatment and has now demonstrated its capacity to develop resistance to the extended-spectrum cephalosporin, ceftriaxone, the last remaining option for first-line empiric treatment of gonorrhea. An era of untreatable gonorrhea may be approaching, which represents an exceedingly serious public health problem. Herein, we review the evolution, origin and spread of antimicrobial resistance and resistance determinants (with a focus on extended-spectrum cephalosporins) in N. gonorrhoeae, detail the current situation regarding verified treatment failures with extended-spectrum cephalosporins and future treatment options, and highlight essential actions to meet the large public health challenge that arises with the possible emergence of untreatable gonorrhea. Essential actions include: implementing action/response plans globally and nationally; enhancing surveillance of gonococcal antimicrobial resistance, treatment failures and antimicrobial use/misuse; and improving prevention, early diagnosis and treatment of gonorrhea. Novel treatment strategies, antimicrobials (or other compounds) and, ideally, a vaccine must be developed."

United States Department of Agriculture. (2011). *Antimicrobial resistance*. USDA Food Safety Research Information Office.
http://www.motherearthnews.com/blogs/~/media/8AFD51289F9843528658597B0F99F324.ashx (cached)

- "Microbial populations acquire AMR through two main mechanisms. These include: Mutation…Gene Transfer…by horizontal gene transfer (HGT) which is mediated by three mechanisms: Transformation, Conjugation and Transduction."
- This article also includes information on "Natural Reservoirs and Transmission,"… "Detection Methods (Antimicrobial Susceptibility Testing),"… "Prevention and Control of Antimicrobial Resistance" and "Foodborne Disease Outbreaks."
- Includes an extensive bibliography.

United States Department of Health & Human Services. (2010). *Antibiotic resistance and the threat to public health.*
http://www.hhs.gov/asl/testify/2010/04/t20100428b.html

- "Antimicrobials are used to treat infections by different disease-causing microorganisms, including bacteria, mycobacteria, viruses, parasites and fungi. In the vast majority of cases where antimicrobials are used, the microorganisms have found a way to evade or resist the antimicrobial agent. Resistance occurs whenever antimicrobials are used – in the community, on the farm, and in healthcare. Antimicrobial resistance is a global problem, and some of our most significant global threats are multi-drug resistant tuberculosis and drug-resistant malaria."

- "The newest resistance challenge in the healthcare setting is multi-drug resistant gram-negative bacteria. Particularly concerning are the carbapenemase-producing bacteria, such as bacteria of the *Klebsiella* species, among others."
- "Antimicrobialis is a general term for the drugs, chemicals, or other substances that wither kill or slow the growth of microbes. Among the antimicrobial agents in use today are antibiotic drugs (which kill bacteria), antiviral agents (which kill viruses), antifungal agents (which kill fungi), and antiparisitic drugs (which kill parasites). An antibiotic is a type of antimicrobial agent made from a mold or a bacterium that kills, or slows the growth of other microbes, specifically bacteria. Examples include penicillin and streptomycin."

Van Boeckel, T. P., Brower, C., Gilbert, M., et al. (2015). Global trends in antimicrobial use in food animals. *Proceedings of the National Academy of Sciences.* 112(18). pg. 5649-54. www.pnas.org/cgi/doi/10.1073/pnas.1503141112

- "Demand for animal protein for human consumption is rising globally at an unprecedented rate…there has been no quantitative measurement of global antimicrobial consumption by livestock."
- "We estimate that the global average annual consumption of antimicrobials per kilogram of animal produced [in] 2010 was 45 mg•kg^{-1}, 148 mg•kg^{-1}, and 172 mg•kg^{-1} for cattle, chicken, and pigs, respectively."
- "For Brazil, Russia, India, China, and South Africa, the increase in antimicrobial consumption will be 99%, [by 2030] up to seven times the projected population growth in this group of countries."
- "This rise is likely to be driven by the growth in consumer demand for livestock products in middle-income countries and a shift to large-scale farms where antimicrobials are used routinely."

Valdez, L., Rêgo, H., Stanley, H. and Braunstein, L. (2015). Predicting the extinction of Ebola spreading in Liberia due to mitigation strategies. *Quantitative Biology.* http://arxiv.org/abs/1502.01326

Van Loon, H. J., Vriens, M. R., Fluit, A. C., et al. (2004). Antibiotic rotation and development of gram-negative antibiotic resistance. *American Journal of Respiratory Critical Care Medicine.* 171(5). pg. 480-87. http://www.atsjournals.org/doi/abs/10.1164/rccm.200401-070OC#.VsigQfkrLmg

- "Cycling of homogeneous antibiotic exposure is unlikely to control the emergence of gram-negative antimicrobial resistance in intensive care units."

Voyles, J., et al. (2014). Moving beyond too little, too late: Managing emerging infectious diseases in wild populations requires international policy and partnerships. *EcoHealth*. https://nature.berkeley.edu/rosenblum/Rosenblum%20Lab%20UC%20Berkeley%20ESPM%20-%20Publications_files/Voyles_EcoHealth_2014.pdf

- "Emerging infectious diseases (EIDs) are on the rise due to multiple factors, including human facilitated movement of pathogens, broad-scale landscape changes, and perturbations to ecological systems (Jones et al. 2008; Fisher et al 2012)."
- "Epidemics in wildlife are problematic because they can lead to pathogen spillover to new host organisms, erode biodiversity and threaten ecosystems that sustain human societies."

Waggoner, J. J., Soda, E. A. and Deresinski, S. (2013). Rare and emerging viral infections in transplant recipients. *Immunocompromised Hosts*. 57(8). pg. 1182-88. http://cid.oxfordjournals.org/content/57/8/1182.full

- "Rare and emerging viruses in the transplant population [include]: human T-cell leukemia virus type 1; hepatitis E virus; bocavirus; KI and WU polyomaviruses; coronaviruses HKU1 and NL63; influenza, H1N1; measles, dengue; rabies; and lymphocytic choriomeningitis virus. Detection and reporting of such rare pathogens in transplant recipients is critical to patient care and improving our understanding of posttransplant infections."

Walker, B., Barrett, S., Polasky, S., et al. (2009). Looming global-scale failures and missing institutions. *Science*. (325). pg. 1345-46. http://www.sciencemag.org/cgi/pmidlookup?view=long&pmid=19745137

Walsh C. (2000). Molecular mechanisms that confer antibacterial drug resistance. *Nature*. 406(6797). pg. 775-81. http://www.ncbi.nlm.nih.gov/pubmed/10963607

Walsh, C. (2003). *Antibiotics: Actions, origins, resistance*. ASM Press, Washington, DC.

Wang, H., et al. (2006). Food commensal microbes as a potentially important avenue in transmitting antibiotic resistance genes. *FEMS Microbiology Letters*. 254. pg. 226-31. http://onlinelibrary.wiley.com/doi/10.1111/j.1574-6968.2005.00030.x/epdf

- "The magnitude of the antibiotic resistance (AR) gene pool in food-borne commensal microbes is yet to be revealed."

- "The presence of 10^2 - 10^7 CFU of ART bacteria per gram of foods in many samples, particularly in ready-to-eat, 'healthy' food items, indicates that the ART bacteria are abundant in the food chain."
- "*Streptococcus thermophiles* was found to be a major host for AR genes in cheese microbiota."
- "The data indicate that food could be an important avenue for ART bacterial evolution and dissemination."
- "Bacterial transmission of AR genes from milk, pork, shrimp, salad ingredients, and numerous cheese types to 'oral residential bacterium' were documented."
- "Oral cavity could be an important area where many initial interactions between food microbes and human microbiota, including horizontal gene transfer events such as conjugation and transformation, might take place during the retention of food residues in the oral cavity."

Wang, L., Chen, Y. P., Miller, K. P., et al. (2014). Functionalised nanoparticles complexed with antibiotic efficiently kill MRSA and other bacteria. *Chem Commun.* 50(81). pg. 12030-3. http://pubs.rsc.org/en/content/articlelanding/2014/cc/c4cc04936e#!divAbstract

Wang, Y. (2006). *Antibiotic-conjugated polyacrylate nanoparticles: New opportunities for development of anti-MRSA agents.* Graduate Theses and Dissertations. http://scholarcommons.usf.edu/cgi/viewcontent.cgi?article=3745&context=etd

Webb, S., Ternes, T., Gibert, M. and Olejniczak, K. (2003). Indirect human exposure to pharmaceuticals via drinking water. *Toxicol Lett.* 142(3). pg. 157–67. http://www.sciencedirect.com/science/article/pii/S0378427403000717

Weintraub, K. (February 16, 2016). New culprit in Lyme disease: Researchers in Minnesota have discovered a new species of tick-borne bacteria. *The New York Times.* pg. D4. http://www.nytimes.com/2016/02/16/health/lyme-disease-cause-bacteria-borrelia-mayonii.html?_r=0

- "The new species, provisionally named Borrelia mayonii, after the clinic, has been found only in the upper Midwest but may be present elsewhere."
- "Available diagnostic screens may be missing others infected with the newly discovered bacteria, the scientists acknowledged."
- "Only one of the six patients had the bull's-eye rash that is Lyme's signature, present in 70 percent to 80 percent of reported cases."

Welch, T. J., Fricke, W. F., McDermott, D. G., et al. (2007). Multiple antimicrobial resistance in plague: an emerging public health risk. *PLOS One.* 3. pg. 1-6. http://journals.plos.org/plosone/article?id=10.1371/journal.pone.0000309

- "*Yersinia pestis*, the etiological agent of plague, is a zoonotic bacterial pathogen that has caused multiple pandemics resulting in an estimated 200 million human deaths."
- "Plague has recently been recognized as a re-emerging disease as small outbreaks continue to occur globally. This reappearance, coupled with its potential for aerosol dissemination and associated high mortality rate, also makes *Y. pestis* one of the most dangerous bioterrorism agents."
- "Plasmid-positive strains were isolated from beef, chicken, turkey and pork, and were found in samples from the following states: California, Colorado, Connecticut, Georgia, Maryland, Minnesota, New Mexico, New York and Oregon…this common plasmid backbone is broadly disseminated among MDB zoonotic pathogens associated with agriculture."

Wellington, E., et al. (2013). The role of the natural environment in the emergence of antibiotic resistance in Gram-negative bacteria. *Lancet: Infectious Disease*. 13(2). pg. 155-65. http://www.ncbi.nlm.nih.gov/pubmed/23347633

- "During the past 10 years, multidrug-resistant Gram-negative Enterobacteriaceae have become a substantial challenge to infection control."
- "The effectiveness of antibiotics is in such rapid decline that, depending on the pathogen concerned, their future utility can be measured in decades or even years. Unless the rise in antibiotic resistance can be reversed, we can expect to see a substantial rise in incurable infection and fatality in both developed and developing regions."
- "The selective effects of pollutants an co-select for mobile genetic elements carrying multiple resistant genes. Anthropogenic activity might be causing evolution of antibiotic resistance in the environment."
- "As the human population increases, and mega cities grow, there is greater risk that infectious diseases will evolve, emerge, or spread readily among the most substantial reservoir of multidrug-resistant Gram-negative bacilli (Enterobacteriaceae and *Pseudomonas aeuginosa*) is the gut of man and animals."
- "CTX-M-a5 is the most widely distributed, having reached endemic prevalence in much of Asia, southern Europe, and South America."
- "The absence of full environmental fate and effect data of antibiotics inhibits an effective assessment of the potential risk through environmental pathways…The future development of more effective biodegradable antibiotics might facilitate their rapid degradation in the environment."

- "The most important emerging public health threats is that of large-scale dissemination of multi-resistant pathogens in the hospital environment, the community, and the wider environment" contributing to a global antibiotic resistance crisis.

Wenzel, R. P. (2004). The antibiotic pipeline-challenges, costs, and values. *New England Journal of Medicine*. 351. pg. 523-6. http://www.nejm.org/doi/pdf/10.1056/NEJMp048093

White, D., et al. (2001). The isolation of antibiotic-resistant salmonella from retail ground meats. *The New England Journal of Medicine*. 345(16). pg. 1147-54. http://www.nejm.org/doi/full/10.1056/NEJMoa010315

- "We identified and characterized strains of salmonella isolated from ground meats purchased in the Washington, D.C. area."
- "Of 200 meat samples, 41 (20 percent) contained salmonella, with a total of 13 serotypes. Eighty-four percent of the isolates were resistant to at least one antibiotic, and 53 percent were resistant to at least three antibiotics. Sixteen percent of the isolates were resistant to ceftriaxone, the drug of choice for treating salmonellosis in children."
- "Resistant strains of salmonella are common in retail ground meats. These findings provide support for the adoption of guidelines for the prudent use of antibiotics in food animals and for a reduction in the number of pathogens present on farms and in slaughterhouses. National surveillance for antimicrobial-resistant salmonella should be extended to include retail meats."

Wikipedia. (2016). *Foodborne illness*.

- "Microbes (if applicable) can pass through the stomach into the intestine via cells lining the intestinal walls and begin to multiply."

Wolfe, N. D., Dunavan, C. P. and Diamond, J. (2007). Origins of major human infectious diseases. *Nature*. 447. pg. 279-83.

Wolska, K. I., Grzes, K. and Kurek, A. (2012). Synergy between novel antimicrobials and conventional antibiotics or bacteriocins. *Polish Journal of Microbiology*. 61(2). pg. 95-104. http://www.pjmonline.org/wp-content/uploads/2015/11/vol6122012095.pdf

Woodford, N., Turton, J. and Livermore, D. (2011). Multiresistant Gram-negative bacteria: The role of high-risk clones in the dissemination of antibiotic resistance. *FEMS Microbiology Review*. 35(5). pg. 736-55. http://femsre.oxfordjournals.org/cgi/pmidlookup?view=long&pmid=21303394

- "'High-risk clones' play a major role in the spread of resistance, with the risk lying in their tenacity – deriving from poorly understood survival traits – and a flexible ability to accumulate and switch resistance, rather than to constant resistance batteries."
- "Limiting the spread of multi-resistant strains is considered to be an infection control priority."

World Health Organization. (2001). *The WHO global strategy of containment of antimicrobial resistance.* World Health Organization. http://www.who.int/drugresistance/WHO_Global_Strategy_English.pdf

World Health Organization. (2012). *The evolving threat of antimicrobial resistance; Options for action.* World Health Organization. http://apps.who.int/iris/bitstream/10665/44812/1/9789241503181_eng.pdf

- "Antimicrobial resistance (AMR) is not a recent phenomenon, but it is a critical health issue today. Over several decades, to varying degrees, bacteria causing common infections have developed resistance to each new antibiotic, and AMR has evolved to become a worldwide health threat. With a dearth of new antibiotics coming to market, the need for action to avert a developing global crisis in health care is increasingly urgent."
- "The use of vast quantities of antibiotics in food-producing animals adds another dimension to a complex situation."
- "Infections which are increasingly resistant to antibiotics together account for a heavy disease burden, often affecting developing countries disproportionately."

World Health Organization. (2012). *Global action plan to control the spread and impact of antimicrobial resistance in Neisseria gonorrhoeae.* Department of Reproductive Health and Research, World Health Organization. http://www.who.int/reproductivehealth/publications/rtis/9789241503501/en/

World Health Organization. (2012). *Global incidence and prevalence of selected curable sexually transmitted infections – 2008.* Department of Reproductive Health and Research, World Health Organization. http://www.who.int/reproductivehealth/publications/rtis/stisestimates/en/

World Health Organization. (2014). *Antimicrobial resistance: Global report on surveillance 2014.* World Health Organization. http://www.who.int/drugresistance/documents/surveillancereport/en/

- "AMR develops when a microorganism (bacteria, fungus, virus or parasite) no longer responds to a drug to which it was originally sensitive."

- "A post-antibiotic era – in which common infections and minor injuries can kill – far from being an apocalyptic fantasy, is instead a very real possibility for the 21st century."
- This WHO report provides as accurate a picture as is presently possible of the magnitude of AMR and the current state of surveillance globally. Very high rates of resistance have been observed in all WHO regions in common bacteria…Overall, surveillance of ABR is neither coordinated nor harmonized."
- Of 194 SHO member states, those providing data on 9 common types of ABR infections ranged from 92 to 35, with 42 nations providing data on ABR gonorrhea.
- "Globally, 3.6% of new TB cases and 20.2% of previously treated cases are estimated to have multidrug-resistant TB (MDR-TB), with much higher rates in Eastern Europe and central Asia…The 84,000 cases of MDR-TB notified to WHO in 2012 represented only about 21% of the MDR-TB cases estimated to have emerged in the world that year."
- "AMR is a global health security threat that requires action across government sectors and society as a whole. Surveillance that generates reliable data is the essential foundation of global strategies and public health actions to contain AMR."

World Health Organization. (2014a). *Tuberculosis in the WHO European region.* World Health Organization. http://www.euro.who.int/__data/assets/pdf_file/0006/244743/Fact-sheet,-Tuberculosis-in-the-WHO-European-Region-Eng.pdf

- "Tuberculosis (TB) continues to be a major public health issue in the WHO European Region. According to the latest estimates, about 360,000 new TB cases and 38,000 deaths were reported in the Region in 2013, mostly from Eastern and central European countries."
- "TB in the Region is becoming more and more difficult to treat…The treatment-success rate for people with multidrug-resistant TB (MDR-TB) was 49% in 2010."
- "Of the 27 countries in the world with a high burden of MDR-TB, 15 are in the WHO European Region: Armenia, Azerbaijan, Belarus, Bulgaria, Estonia, Georgia, Kazakhstan, Kyrgyzstan, Latvia, Lithuania, the Republic of Moldova, the Russian Federation, Tajikistan, Ukraine and Uzbekistan. A recent study shows that the Region has the highest rate documented in the world of MDR-TB among new cases (35%) and previously treated cases (69%). Around 76,400 people in the WHO European Region are estimated to fall sick with MDR-TB

every year. Owing to limited access to diagnosis, only 33,400 (44%) of them were diagnosed in 2012. While almost all MDR-TB patients now have access to treatment, the rate of successful treatment is below the 75% target."

- "MDR-TB is resistant to two of the most potent anti-TB drugs. It is a man-made phenomenon that emerged as a result of inadequate treatment of TB and/or poor airborne infection control in health care facilities and congregate settings. XDR-TB is resistant to the most important first- and second-line drugs and has very limited chances for cure."

World Health Organization. (2014b). *WHO's first global report on antibiotic resistance reveals serious, worldwide threat to public health*. World Health Organization. http://www.who.int/mediacentre/news/releases/2014/amr-report/en/.

- "Antibiotic resistance-when bacteria change so antibiotics no longer work in people who need them to treat infections-is now a major threat to public health."
- "Effective antibiotics have been one of the pillars allowing us to live longer, live healthier, and benefit from modern medicine. Unless we take significant actions to improve efforts to prevent infections and also change how we produce, prescribe and use antibiotics, the world will lose more and more of these global public health goods and the implications will be devastating."

World Health Organization. (2015a). *Global tuberculosis report, 2015*. World Health Organization.
http://apps.who.int/iris/bitstream/10665/191102/1/9789241565059_eng.pdf?ua=1

World Health Organization. (2015b). *Multidrug-resistant tuberculosis (MDR-TB): 2015 update*. WHO. http://www.who.int/tb/challenges/mdr/mdr_tb_factsheet.pdf?ua=1

Wright, G. (2005). Bacterial resistance to antibiotics: Enzymatic degradation and modification. *Advanced Drug Delivery Reviews*. 57(10). pg. 1451-70. http://www.ncbi.nlm.nih.gov/pubmed/15950313

- "A unique feature of enzymes that physically modify antibiotics is that these mechanisms alone actively reduce the concentration of drugs in the local environment; therefore, they present a unique challenge to researchers and clinicians considering new approaches to anti-infective therapy...A thorough understanding of resistance enzyme molecular mechanism, three-dimensional structure, and evolution can be leveraged in combating resistance."
- "Given the fact that the antibiotic drug discovery pipeline is going dry, creative leverage of the understanding of the details of enzyme-based resistance has a significant impact on the treatment of infectious diseases."

Wright, M., Peltier, G., Stepanauskas, R. and McArthur, J. (2006). Bacterial tolerances to metals and antibiotics in metal-contaminated and reference streams. *FEMS Microbiology and Ecology*. 58(2). pg. 293-302. http://www.ncbi.nlm.nih.gov/pubmed/17064270

Wright, M., Baker-Austin, C., Lindell, A., et al. (2008). Influence of industrial contamination on mobile genetic elements: Class 1 integron abundance and gene cassette structure in aquatic bacterial communities. *International Society for Microbial Ecology Journal*. 2(4). pg. 417-28. http://www.ncbi.nlm.nih.gov/pubmed/18273063

Xi, C., et al. (2009). Prevalence of antibiotic resistance in drinking water treatment and distribution systems. *Applied and Environmental Microbiology*. 75(17). pg. 5714-8. http://aem.asm.org/content/75/17/5714.full

- "Aquatic ecosystems are a recognized reservoir for ARB (antibiotic-resistant bacteria. We used culture-dependent methods and quantitative molecular techniques to detect and quantify ARB and antibiotic resistance genes (ARGs) in source waters, drinking water treatment plants, and tap water from several cities in Michigan and Ohio"
- "We found ARGs and heterotrophic ARB in all finished water and tap water tested, although the amounts were small. The quantities of most ARGs were greater in tap water than in finished water and source water."
- In general, the levels of bacteria were higher in source water than in tap water, and the levels of ARB were higher in tap water than in finished water, indicating that there was regrowth of bacteria in drinking water distribution systems."
- "Elevated resistance to some antibiotics was observed during water treatment and in tap water. Water treatment might increase the antibiotic resistance of surviving bacteria, and water distribution systems may serve as an important reservoir for the spread of antibiotic resistance to opportunistic pathogens."

Yan, M., Pamp, S., Fukuyama, J., et al. (2014). Nasal microenvironments and interspecific interactions influence nasal microbiota complexity and S. aureus carriage. *Cell Host Microbe*. 14(6). pg. 631-40. http://www.ncbi.nlm.nih.gov/pmc/articles/PMC3902146/

- "The indigenous microbiota of the nasal cavity plays important roles in human health and disease. Patterns of spatial variation in microbiota composition may help explain Staphylococcus aureus colonization and reveal interspecies and species-host interactions. To assess the biogeography of the nasal microbiota, we sampled healthy subjects, representing both S. aureus carriers and noncarriers at three nasal sites (anterior naris, middle meatus, and sphenoethmoidal recess).

Phylogenetic compositional and sparse linear discriminant analyses revealed communities that differed according to site epithelium type and S. aureus culture-based carriage status. Corynebacterium accolens and C. pseudodiphtheriticum were identified as the most important microbial community determinants of S. aureus carriage, and competitive interactions were only evident at sites with ciliated pseudostratified columnar epithelium. In vitro cocultivation experiments provided supporting evidence of interactions among these species. These results highlight spatial variation in nasal microbial communities and differences in community composition between S. aureus carriers and noncarriers."

Yang, S.W. and Carlson, K. (2003). Evolution of antibiotic occurrence in a river through pristine, urban and agricultural landscapes. *Water Research*. 37(19). pg. 4645-56.

Yoshikawa, T. T. (2002). Antimicrobial resistance and aging: Beginning of the end of the Antibiotic Era. *Journal of the American Geriatrics Society*. 50(s7). pg. S226-9. http://onlinelibrary.wiley.com/doi/10.1046/j.1532-5415.50.7s.2.x/abstract

- "The large volume of antibiotics prescribed has contributed to the emergence of highly resistant pathogens among geriatric patients…Unless preventive strategies coupled with newer drug development are established soon, eventually clinicians will be encountering infections caused by highly resistant pathogens for which no effective antibiotics will be available."

Zetola, N., et al. (2005). Community-acquired methicillin-resistant *Staphylococcus aureus*: An emerging threat. *Lancet Infectious Disease*. 5(5). pg. 275-86. http://www.ncbi.nlm.nih.gov/pubmed/15854883

- "Outbreaks of epidemic furunculosis and cases of severe invasive pulmonary infections in young, otherwise healthy people have been particularly noteworthy…New strains of community-acquired MRSA have contributed to their pathogenicity."

Zhang, R., Eggleston, K., Rotimi, V. and Zeckhauser, R. J. (2006). Antibiotic resistance as a global threat: evidence from China, Kuwait and the United States. *Globalization and Health*. 2(6). pg. 1-14. http://www.globalizationandhealth.com/content/2/1/6.

- "We find that China has the highest level of antibiotic resistance, followed by Kuwait and the U.S…China also has the most rapid growth rate of resistance (22% average growth in a study spanning 1994 to 2000)."

- "Antimicrobial resistance is a serious and growing problem in all three countries. To date, there is no strong international convergence in the countries' resistance patterns. This finding may change with the greater international travel that will accompany globalization. Future research on the determinants of drug resistance patterns, and their international convergence or divergence, should be a priority."

Zhang, X., Zhang, T. and Fang, H. (2009). Antibiotic resistance genes in water environment. *Applied Microbiology and Biotechnology*. 82. pg. 397-414. https://www.researchgate.net/publication/23764846_Antibiotic_resistant_genes_in_water_environment

- "The majority of antibiotics are excreted unchanged into the environment."
- "Hundreds of various ARGs encoding resistance to a broad range of antibiotics have been found in microorganisms distributed not only in hospital wastewaters and animal production wastewaters, but also in sewage, wastewater treatment plants, surface water, groundwater, and even in drinking water."
- "Applications of antibiotics in human, veterinary medicine, and agriculture for nearly 60 years have exerted a major impact on bacterial communities, resulting in…hundreds of ARGs being detected in various water environments."
- "In Europe, nearly all types of ARGs were frequently detected in aquatic environments of some countries, including Germany, Portugal, Belgium, Denmark and Greece…As a result of extensive use of human and veterinary antibiotics, hospital wastewater and livestock manure are considered as the major sources of environmental ARGs."
- "Vancomycin resistance genes have been detected in dairy farm water of Italy, human-derived wastewater of England, urban raw sewage, treated sewage and surface water of Sweden [and] municipal wastewater, surface water, and drinking water biofilms of Germany."
- "ARGs can be transferred into soils by amending farm land with animal manure and processed biosludge from STPs and then can leach to groundwater or be carried by runoff and erosion to surface water."
- "Surface water and shallow groundwater are commonly used as source of drinking water; thus, ARGs can go through drinking water treatment facilities and enter into water distribution systems."
- "Sewage receives the bacteria previously exposed to antibiotics from private households and hospitals and is considered as a hotspot for ARGs. ARGs go into STPs with sewage water, and most of them cannot be effectively removed with traditional treatment process before being released into the environments."

- "STP effluent and sludge application to agricultural fields are recognized as important sources of ARGs to surface waters and soils and subsequently into groundwater."
- "ARgs emerge in aquatic environments as a direct result of intensive use of antibiotics in hospitals, swine production areas, and fish farms."
- "ARGs themselves could be considered as environmental 'pollutants' since they are widely distributed in various environmental compartments, including wastewater and STPs, surface water, lagoon water of animal production areas, aquaculture water, sediments and soil, groundwater, and drinking water."

Zhang, Y., Marrs, C., Simon, C. and Xi, C. (2009).Wastewater treatment contributes to selective increase of antibiotic resistance among Acinetobacter spp. *Science of the Total Environment*. 407. pg. 3702-6. http://graham.umich.edu/media/pubs/zhang-article.pdf

Zhou, Q., Luo, Y. and Wang, M. (2007). Environmental residues and ecotoxicity of antibiotics and their resistance gene pollution: A review. *Asian Journal of Ecotoxicology*. 2. pg. 243-51. http://en.cnki.com.cn/Article_en/CJFDTotal-STDL200703001.htm

Zignol, M., et al. (2006). Global incidence of multidrug-resistant tuberculosis. *Journal of Infectious Diseases*. 194(4). pg. 479-85. http://jid.oxfordjournals.org/content/194/4/479.full

- "The total number of MDR-TB cases estimated to have occurred worldwide in 2004 is 424,203 or 4.3% of all new and previously treated TB cases."
- "In the same year, 181,408 MDR-TB cases were estimated to have occurred among previously treated TB cases alone."
- "Three countries – China, India, and the Russian Federation – accounted for 261,362 MDR-TB cases, or 62% of the estimated global burden."

Zinner, Stephen. (1999). Changing epidemiology of infections in patients with Neutropenia and Cancer: emphasis on Gram-positive and Resistant bacteria. *Clinical Infectious Diseases*. 29. pg. 490-94. http://cid.oxfordjournals.org/content/29/3/490.full.pdf

- "Twenty years ago [1979], gram-negative bacteria caused ~70% of bloodstream infections."
- "In most centers today, ~70% of bacteremic isolates are gram-positive cocci…Gram-positive organisms are becoming increasingly frequent in patients with neutropenia."
- "Several 'new' organisms…now cause infections in these patients."

Appendix 1: Centers for Disease Control: Antibiotic Resistance: Threats in the United States, 2013

Table of Contents

106

Foreward

Antimicrobial resistance is one of our most serious health threats. Infections from resistant bacteria are now too common, and some pathogens have even become resistant to multiple types or classes of antibiotics (antimicrobials used to treat bacterial infections).The loss of effective antibiotics will undermine our ability to fight infectious diseases and manage the infectious complications common in vulnerable patients undergoing chemotherapy for cancer, dialysis for renal failure, and surgery, especially organ transplantation, for which the ability to treat secondary infections is crucial.

When first-line and then second-line antibiotic treatment options are limited by resistance or are unavailable, healthcare providers are forced to use antibiotics that may be more toxic to the patient and frequently more expensive and less effective. Even when alternative treatments exist, research has shown that patients with resistant infections are often much more likely to die, and survivors have significantly longer hospital stays, delayed recuperation, and long-term disability. Efforts to prevent such threats build on the foundation of proven public health strategies: immunization, infection control, protecting the food supply, antibiotic stewardship, and reducing person-to-person spread through screening, treatment and education.

Dr.Tom Frieden, MD, MPH

Director, U.S. Centers for Disease Control and Prevention

Meeting the Challenges of Drug-Resistant Diseases in Developing Countries

Committee on Foreign Affairs Subcommittee on Africa, Global Health, Human Rights, and International Organizations

United States House of Representatives

April 23, 2013

Antibiotic Resistance Threats in the United States, 2013

Executive Summary

Antibiotic Resistance Threats in the United States, 2013 is a snapshot of the complex problem of antibiotic resistance today and the potentially catastrophic consequences of inaction. The overriding purpose of this report is to increase awareness of the threat that antibiotic resistance poses and to encourage immediate action to address the threat. This document can serve as a reference for anyone looking for information about antibiotic resistance. It is specifically designed to be accessible to many audiences. For more technical information, references and links are provided.

This report covers bacteria causing severe human infections and the antibiotics used to treat those infections. In addition, *Candida,* a fungus that commonly causes serious illness, especially among hospital patients, is included because it, too, is showing increasing resistance to the drugs used for treatment. When discussing the pathogens included in this report, *Candida* will be included when referencing "bacteria" for simplicity. Also, infections caused by the bacteria *Clostridium difficile (C. difficile)* are also included in this report. Although *C. difficile* infections are not yet significantly resistant to the drugs used to treat them, most are directly related to antibiotic use and thousands of Americans are affected each year.

Drug resistance related to viruses such as HIV and influenza is not included, nor is drug resistance among parasites such as those that cause malaria. These are important problems but are beyond the scope of this report. The report consists of multiple one or two page summaries of cross-cutting and bacteria- specific antibiotic resistance topics. The first section provides context and an overview of antibiotic resistance in the United States. In addition to giving a national assessment of the most dangerous antibiotic resistance threats, it summarizes what is known about the burden of illness, level of concern, and antibiotics left to defend against these infections. This first section also includes some basic background information, such as fact sheets about antibiotic safety and the harmful impact that resistance can have on high-risk groups, including those with chronic illnesses such as cancer.

CDC estimates that in the United States, more than two million people are sickened every year with antibiotic-resistant infections, with at least 23,000 dying as a result. The estimates are based on conservative assumptions and are likely minimum estimates. They are the best approximations that can be derived from currently available data.

Regarding level of concern, CDC has — for the first time — prioritized bacteria in this report into one of three categories: urgent, serious, and concerning.

Urgent Threats

Clostridium difficile

Carbapenem-resistant Enterobacteriaceae (CRE)

Drug-resistant *Neisseria gonorrhoeae*

Serious Threats

Multidrug-resistant *Acinetobacter*

Drug-resistant *Campylobacter*

Fluconazole-resistant *Candida* (a fungus)

Extended spectrum β-lactamase producing Enterobacteriaceae (ESBLs)

Vancomycin-resistant *Enterococcus* (VRE)

Multidrug-resistant *Pseudomonas aeruginosa*

Drug-resistant Non-typhoidal *Salmonella*

Drug-resistant *Salmonella* Typhi

Drug-resistant *Shigella*

Methicillin-resistant *Staphylococcus aureus* (MRSA)

Drug-resistant *Streptococcus pneumoniae*

Drug-resistant tuberculosis

Concerning Threats

Vancomycin-resistant *Staphylococcus aureus* (VRSA)

Erythromycin-resistant Group A *Streptococcus*

Clindamycin-resistant Group B *Streptococcus*

The second section describes what can be done to combat this growing threat, including information on current CDC initiatives. Four core actions that fight the spread of antibiotic resistance are presented and explained, including 1) preventing infections from occurring and preventing resistant bacteria from spreading, 2) tracking resistant bacteria, 3) improving the use of antibiotics, and 4) promoting the development of new antibiotics and new diagnostic tests for resistant bacteria.

The third section provides summaries of each of the bacteria in this report. These summaries can aid in discussions about each bacteria, how to manage infections, and implications for public health. They also highlight the similarities and differences among the many different types of infections.

This section also includes information about what groups such as states, communities, doctors, nurses, patients, and CDC can do to combat antibiotic resistance. Preventing the spread of antibiotic resistance can only be achieved with widespread engagement, especially among leaders in clinical medicine, healthcare leadership, agriculture, and public health. Although some people are at greater risk than others, no one can completely avoid the risk of antibiotic-resistant infections. Only through concerted commitment and action will the nation ever be able to succeed in reducing this threat.

A reference section provides technical information, a glossary, and additional resources.

Any comments and suggestions that would improve the usefulness of future publications are appreciated and should be sent to Director, Division of Healthcare Quality Promotion, National Center for Emerging and Zoonotic Infectious Diseases, Centers for Disease Control and Prevention, 1600 Clifton Road, Mailstop A-07, Atlanta, Georgia, 30333.E-mail can also be used: hip@cdc.gov.

The Threat of Antibiotic Resistance

Introduction

Antibiotic resistance is a worldwide problem. New forms of antibiotic resistance can cross international boundaries and spread between continents with ease. Many forms of resistance spread with remarkable speed. World health leaders have described antibiotic-resistant microorganisms as "nightmare bacteria" that "pose a catastrophic threat" to people in every country in the world.

Each year in the United States, at least 2 million people acquire serious infections with bacteria that are resistant to one or more of the antibiotics designed to treat those infections. At least 23,000 people die each year as a direct result of these antibiotic-resistant infections. Many more die from other conditions that were complicated by an antibiotic-resistant infection.

In addition, almost 250,000 people each year require hospital care for *Clostridium difficile (C. difficile)* infections. In most of these infections, the use of antibiotics was a major contributing factor leading to the illness. At least 14,000 people die each year in the United States from *C. difficile* infections. Many of these infections could have been prevented.

Antibiotic-resistant infections add considerable and avoidable costs to the already overburdened U.S. healthcare system. In most cases, antibiotic-resistant infections require prolonged and/or costlier treatments, extend hospital stays, necessitate additional doctor visits and healthcare use, and result in greater disability and death compared with infections that are easily treatable with antibiotics. The total economic cost of antibiotic resistance to the U.S. economy has been difficult to calculate. Estimates vary but have ranged as high as $20 billion in excess direct healthcare costs, with additional costs to society for lost productivity as high as $35 billion a year (2008 dollars).[1]

The use of antibiotics is the single most important factor leading to antibiotic resistance around the world. Antibiotics are among the most commonly prescribed drugs used in human medicine. However, up to 50% of all the antibiotics prescribed for people are not needed or are not optimally effective as prescribed. Antibiotics are also commonly used in food animals to prevent, control, and treat disease, and to promote the growth of food-producing animals. The use of antibiotics for promoting growth is not necessary, and the practice should be phased out. Recent guidance from the U.S. Food and Drug Administration (FDA) describes a pathway toward this goal.[2] It is difficult to directly compare the amount of drugs used in food animals with the amount used in humans, but there is evidence that more antibiotics are used in food production.

The other major factor in the growth of antibiotic resistance is spread of the resistant strains of bacteria from person to person, or from the non-human sources in the environment, including food.

There are four core actions that will help fight these deadly infections:

110

- preventing infections and preventing the spread of resistance
- tracking resistant bacteria
- improving the use of today's antibiotics
- promoting the development of new antibiotics and developing new diagnostic tests for resistant bacteria

Bacteria will inevitably find ways of resisting the antibiotics we develop, which is why aggressive action is needed now to keep new resistance from developing and to prevent the resistance that already exists from spreading.

1 http://www.tufts.edu/med/apua/consumers/personal_home_5_1451036133.pdf (accessed 8-5-2013); extrapolated from Roberts RR, Hota B, Ahmad I, et al. Hospital and societal costs of antimicrobial-resistant infections in a Chicago teaching hospital: implications for antibiotic stewardship. Clin Infect Dis.2009 Oct 15;49(8):1175-84
2 http://www.fda.gov/downloads/AnimalVeterinary/GuidanceComplianceEnforcement/GuidanceforIndustry/UCM2996 24.pdf

National Summary Data

Estimated minimum number of illnesses and deaths caused by antibiotic resistance, including bacteria and fungus: **At least 2,049,442 illnesses and 23,000 deaths**

Estimated minimum number of illnesses and death due to *Clostridium difficile (C. difficile)*, a unique bacterial infection that, although not significantly resistant to the drugs used to treat it, is directly related to antibiotic use and resistance: **At least 250,000 illnesses and 14,000 deaths**

Where do infections happen?

Antibiotic-resistant infections can happen anywhere. Data show that most happen in the general community; however, most deaths related to antibiotic resistance happen in healthcare settings, such as hospitals and nursing homes.

How Antibiotic Resistance Happens

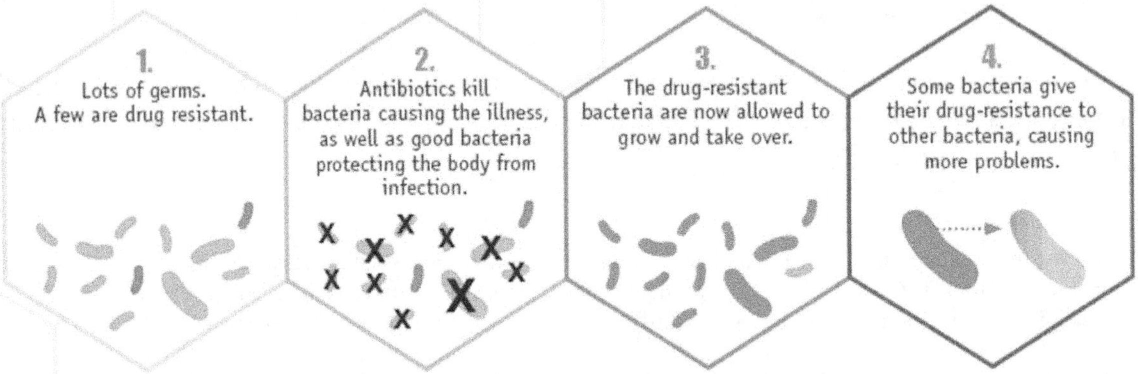

1.
Lots of germs.
A few are drug resistant.

2.
Antibiotics kill bacteria causing the illness, as well as good bacteria protecting the body from infection.

3.
The drug-resistant bacteria are now allowed to grow and take over.

4.
Some bacteria give their drug-resistance to other bacteria, causing more problems.

Examples of How Antibiotic Resistance Spreads

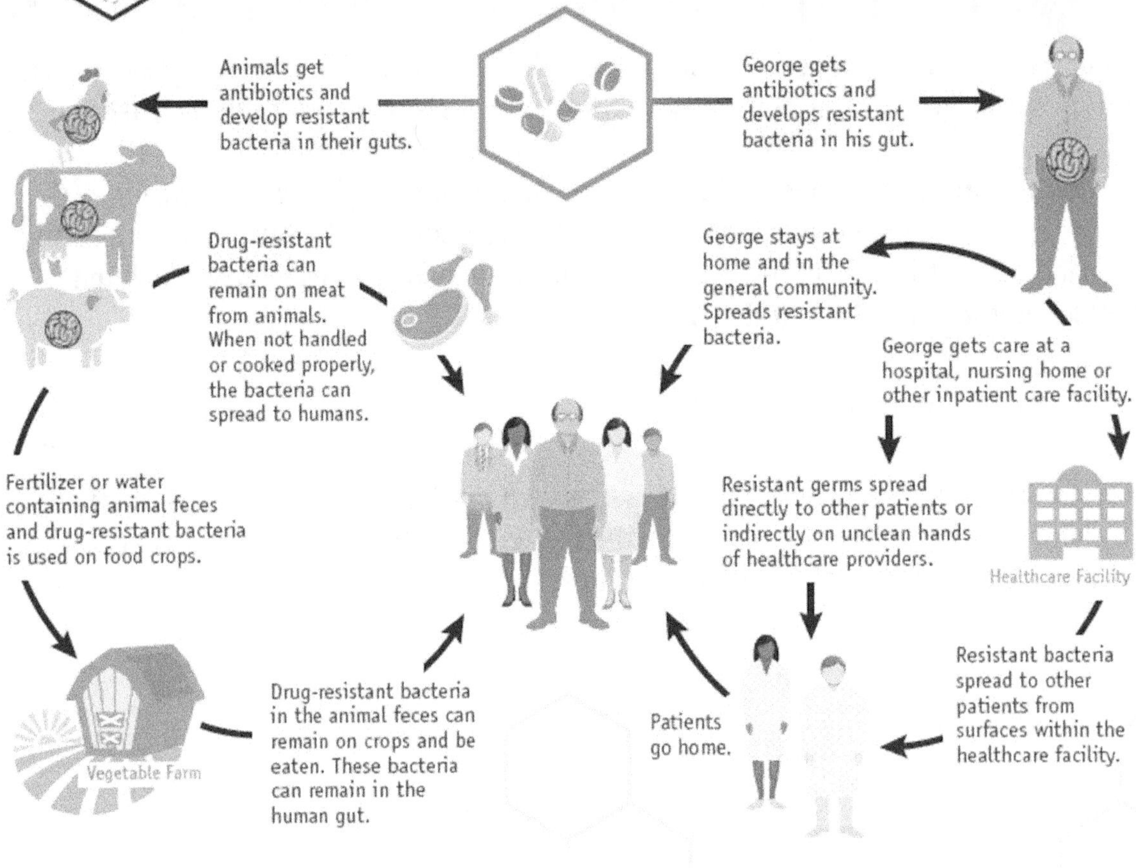

Animals get antibiotics and develop resistant bacteria in their guts.

George gets antibiotics and develops resistant bacteria in his gut.

Drug-resistant bacteria can remain on meat from animals. When not handled or cooked properly, the bacteria can spread to humans.

George stays at home and in the general community. Spreads resistant bacteria.

George gets care at a hospital, nursing home or other inpatient care facility.

Fertilizer or water containing animal feces and drug-resistant bacteria is used on food crops.

Resistant germs spread directly to other patients or indirectly on unclean hands of healthcare providers.

Healthcare Facility

Drug-resistant bacteria in the animal feces can remain on crops and be eaten. These bacteria can remain in the human gut.

Patients go home.

Resistant bacteria spread to other patients from surfaces within the healthcare facility.

Vegetable Farm

Simply using antibiotics creates resistance. These drugs should only be used to treat infections.

Minimum Estimates of Morbidity and Mortality from Antibiotic-Resistant Infections*

Antibiotic-Resistant Microorganism	Infections Included in Case/Death Estimates	Infections Not Included	Estimated Annual Number of Cases	Estimated Annual Number of Deaths
Carbapenem-resistant Enterobacteriaceae (CRE)	Healthcare-associated Infections (HAIs) caused by *Klebsiella* and *E. coli* with onset in hospitalized patients	Infections occurring outside of acute care hospitals (e.g., nursing homes) Infections acquired in acute care hospitals but not diagnosed until after discharge Infections caused by Enterobacteriaceae other than *Klebsiella* and *E. coli* (e.g., *Enterobacter spp.*)	9,300	610
Drug-resistant *Neisseria gonorrhoeae* (any drug)	All infections	Not applicable	246,000	<5
Multidrug-resistant *Acinetobacter* (three or more drug classes)	HAIs with onset in hospitalized patients	Infections occurring outside of acute care hospitals (e.g., nursing homes) Infections acquired in acute care hospitals but not diagnosed until after discharge	7,300	500
Drug-resistant *Campylobacter* (azithromycin or ciprofloxacin)	All infections	Not applicable	310,000	28
Drug-resistant *Candida* (fluconazole)	HAIs with onset in hospitalized patients	Infections occurring outside of acute care hospitals (e.g., nursing homes) Infections acquired in acute care hospitals but not diagnosed until after discharge	3,400	220
Extended-spectrum β-lactamase producing Enterobacteriaceae (ESBLs)	HAIs caused by *Klebsiella* and *E. coli* with onset in hospitalized patients	Infections occurring outside of acute care hospitals (e.g., nursing homes) Infections acquired in acute care hospitals but not diagnosed until after discharge Infections caused by Enterobacteriaceae other than *Klebsiella* and *E. coli* (e.g., Enterobacter *spp.*)	26,000	1,700

113

Antibiotic-Resistant Microorganism	Infections Included in Case/Death Estimates	Infections Not Included	Estimated Annual Number of Cases	Estimated Annual Number of Deaths
Vancomycin-resistant Enterococcus (VRE)	HAIs with onset in hospitalized patients	Infections occurring outside of acute care hospitals (e.g., nursing homes) Infections acquired in acute care hospitals but not diagnosed until after discharge	20,000	1,300
Multidrug-resistant Pseudomonas aeruginosa (three or more drug classes)	HAIs with onset in hospitalized patients	Infections occurring outside of acute care hospitals (e.g., nursing homes) Infections acquired in acute care hospitals but not diagnosed until after discharge	6,700	440
Drug-resistant non-typhoidal Salmonella (ceftriaxone, ciprofloxacin†, or 5 or more drug classes)	All infections	Not applicable	100,000	40
Drug-resistant Salmonella Typhi (ciprofloxacin†)	All infections	Not applicable	3,800	<5
Drug-resistant Shigella (azithromycin or ciprofloxacin)	All infections	Not applicable	27,000	<5
Methicillin-resistant Staphylococcus aureus (MRSA)	Invasive infections	Both healthcare and community-associated non-invasive infections such as wound and skin and soft tissue infections	80,000	11,000
Streptococcus pneumoniae (full resistance to clinically relevant drugs)	All infections	Not applicable	1,200,000	7,000

Antibiotic-Resistant Microorganism	Infections Included in Case/Death Estimates	Infections Not Included	Estimated Annual Number of Cases	Estimated Annual Number of Deaths
Drug-resistant tuberculosis (any clinically relevant drug)	All infections	Not applicable	1,042	50
Vancomycin-resistant *Staphylococcus aureus* (VRSA)	All infections	Not applicable	<5	<5
Erythromycin-resistant Group A *Streptococcus*	Invasive infections	Non-invasive infections including common upper-respiratory infections like strep throat	1,300	160
Clindamycin-resistant Group B *Streptococcus*	Invasive infections	Non-invasive infections and asymptomatic intrapartum colonization requiring prophylaxis	7,600	440
Summary Totals for Antibiotic-Resistant Infections			2,049,442	23,488
Clostridium difficile Infections	Healthcare-associated infections in acute care hospitals or in patients requiring hospitalization	Infections occurring outside of acute care hospitals (e.g. nursing homes, community) Infections acquired in acute care hospitals but not diagnosed until after discharge	250,000	14,000

*See technical appendix for discussion of estimation methods.

†Resistance or partial resistance

115

Limitations of Estimating the Burden of Disease Associated with Antibiotic- Resistant Bacteria

This report uses several methods, described in the technical appendix, to estimate the number of cases of disease caused by antibiotic-resistant bacteria and fungi and the number of deaths resulting from those cases of disease. The data presented in this report are approximations, and totals, as provided in the national summary tables, can provide only a rough estimate of the true burden of illness. Greater precision is not possible at this time for a number of reasons:

- Precise criteria exist for determining the resistance of a particular species of bacteria to a specific antibiotic. However, for many species of bacteria, there are no standard definitions that allow for neatly dividing most species into only two categories—resistant vs. susceptible without regard to a specific antibiotic. This report specifies how resistance is defined for each microorganism.

- There are very specific criteria and algorithms for the attribution of deaths to specific causes that are used for reporting vital statistics data. In general, there are no similar criteria for making clinical determinations of when someone's death is primarily attributable to infection with antibiotic-resistant bacteria, as opposed to other co-existing illnesses that may have contributed to or caused death. Many studies attempting to determine attributable mortality rely on the judgment of chart reviewers, as is the case for many surveillance systems. Thus, the distinction between an antibiotic-resistant infection leading directly to death, an antibiotic-resistant infection contributing to a death, and an antibiotic-resistant infection related to, but not directly contributing to a death are usually determined subjectively, especially in the preponderance of cases where patients are hospitalized and have complicated clinical presentations.

In addition, the estimates provided in this report represent an underestimate of the total burden of bacterial resistant disease.

- The methodology employed in this report likely underestimates, at least for some pathogens, the impact of antibiotic resistance on mortality. As described in the technical appendix, the percentage of resistant isolates for some bacteria was multiplied by the total number of cases or the number of deaths ascribed to that bacterium. A number of studies have shown that the risk of death following infection with a strain of resistant bacteria is greater than that following infection

116

with a susceptible strain of the same bacteria. More accurate data for all bacteria would be necessary to estimate the extent of the differential risk for death associated with a resistant infection vs. the risk of death associated with a susceptible infection. But, lacking that data, the lower, more conservative estimate has been used. That estimate is the approximation of the number of deaths derived by applying the proportion of resistant isolates to the estimated total number of deaths caused by that pathogen.

- For several pathogens, complete data from all types of infections are not available since tracking is limited to the more severe types of infections. For some pathogens, such as methicillin-resistant *Staphylococcus aureus* (MRSA), only cases due to invasive disease are counted. For other pathogens, where resistance is predominately limited to healthcare settings, only disease occurring in acute care hospitals, or requiring hospitalization, are counted.

The actual number of infections and the actual number of deaths, therefore, are certainly higher than the numbers provided in this report.

This report does not provide a specific estimate for the financial cost of antibiotic-resistant infections. Although a variety of studies have attempted to estimate costs in limited settings, such as a single hospital or group of hospitals, the methods used are quite variable. Similarly, careful work has been done to estimate costs for specific pathogens, such as *Streptococcus pneumoniae* and MRSA. However, no consensus methodology currently exists for making such monetary estimates for many of the other pathogens listed in this report. For this reason, this report references non-CDC estimates in the introduction, but does not attempt to estimate the overall financial burden of antibiotic resistance to the United States.

Assessment of Domestic Antibiotic Resistance Threats

CDC conducted an assessment of antibiotic resistance threats, categorizing the threat level of each bacteria as urgent, serious, or concerning. The assessment was done in consultation with non-governmental experts in antibiotic resistance who serve on the Antimicrobial Resistance Working Group of the CDC Office of Infectious Diseases Board of Scientific Counselors (http://www.cdc.gov/oid/BSC.html).CDC also received input and recommendations from the National Institutes of Health (NIH) and the U.S. Food and Drug Administration (FDA).Threats were assessed according to seven factors associated with resistant infections:

- clinical impact

- economic impact
- incidence
- 10-year projection of incidence
- transmissibility
- availability of effective antibiotics
- barriers to prevention

The assessment was focused on domestic impact, but the threat of importing international antibiotic-resistant pathogens was taken into account in the 10-year incidence projection. Because antibiotic resistance is a rapidly evolving problem, this assessment will be revised at least every five years. Examples of findings that could result in a change in threat status are:

- Multidrug-resistant and extensively drug-resistant tuberculosis (MDR and XDR TB) infections are an increasing threat outside of the United States. In the United States, infections are uncommon because a robust prevention and control program is in place. If infection rates of MDR and XDR TB increase within the U.S., this antibiotic-resistant threat will change from serious to urgent, because it is transmissible through respiratory secretions, and because treatment options are very limited.

- MRSA infections can be very serious and the number of infections is among the highest of all antibiotic-resistant threats. However, the number of serious infections is decreasing and there are multiple effective antibiotics for treating infections. If MRSA infection rates increase or MRSA strains become more resistant to other antibiotic agents, then MRSA may change from a serious to an urgent threat.

- *Streptococcus pneumoniae* (pneumococcus) can cause serious and sometimes life-threatening infections. Antibiotic resistance significantly affects the ability to manage these infections. A new version of the pneumococcal conjugate vaccine (PCV13), introduced in 2010, protects against infections with the most resistant pneumococcus strains and rates of resistant infections are declining. The extent to which this trend will continue is unknown, but a significant and sustainable drop in resistant infection rates could result in this threat being recategorized as concerning.

In general, threats assigned to the urgent and serious categories require more monitoring and prevention activities, whereas the threats in the concerning category require less. Regardless of category, threat-specific CDC activities are tailored to meet the epidemiology of the infectious agent and to address any gaps in the ability to detect resistance and to protect against infections.

HAZARD LEVEL
URGENT

⊖ ⊖ ⊖ ⊖ ⊖

These are high-consequence antibiotic-resistant threats because of significant risks identified across several criteria. These threats may not be currently widespread but have the potential to become so and require urgent public health attention to identify infections and to limit transmission.

Clostridium difficile (C. difficile), Carbapenem-resistant Enterobacteriaceae (CRE), Drug-resistant *Neisseria gonorrhoeae* (cephalosporin resistance)

HAZARD LEVEL
SERIOUS

⊖ ⊖ ⊖ ⊖ ⊖

These are significant antibiotic-resistant threats. For varying reasons (e.g., low or declining domestic incidence or reasonable availability of therapeutic agents), they are not considered urgent, but these threats will worsen and may become urgent without ongoing public health monitoring and prevention activities.

Multidrug-resistant *Acinetobacter*, Drug-resistant *Campylobacter*, Fluconazole-resistant *Candida* (a fungus), Extended spectrum β-lactamase producing Enterobacteriaceae (ESBLs), Vancomycin-resistant *Enterococcus* (VRE), Multidrug-resistant *Pseudomonas aeruginosa*, Drug-resistant Non-typhoidal *Salmonella*, Drug-resistant *Salmonella* Typhi, Drug-resistant *Shigella*, Methicillin-resistant *Staphylococcus aureus* (MRSA), Drug-resistant *Streptococcus pneumonia*, Drug-resistant tuberculosis (MDR and XDR)

HAZARD LEVEL
CONCERNING

⊖ ⊖ ⊖ ⊖ ⊖

These are bacteria for which the threat of antibiotic resistance is low, and/ or there are multiple therapeutic options for resistant infections. These bacterial pathogens cause severe illness. Threats in this category require monitoring and in some cases rapid incident or outbreak response.

Vancomycin-resistant *Staphylococcus aureus* (VRSA), Erythromycin-resistant *Streptococcus* Group A, Clindamycin-resistant *Streptococcus* Group B

Although *C. difficile* is not currently significantly resistant to antibiotics used to treat it, it was included in the threat assessment because of its unique relationship with resistance issues, antibiotic use, and its high morbidity and mortality.

119

Running Out of Drugs to Treat Serious Gram-Negative Infections

Among all of the bacterial resistance problems, gram-negative pathogens are particularly worrisome, because they are becoming resistant to nearly all drugs that would be considered for treatment. This is true as well, but not to the same extent, for some of the gram-positive infections (e.g., *Staphylococcus* and *Enterococcus)*. The most serious gram-negative infections are healthcare-associated, and the most common pathogens are Enterobacteriaceae, *Pseudomonas aeruginosa,* and *Acinetobacter*. Treating infections of either pan-resistant or nearly pan-resistant gram-negative microorganisms is an increasingly common challenge in many hospitals. The table below describes the drug classes used to treat these infections and a description of important drug resistance and other limitations. The classes are in order of most likely to be used to less likely to be used.

Drug Class	Important Characteristics	Resistance and Other Limitations
β-lactams	A large class of broad-spectrum drugs that are the main treatment for gram-negative infections. The subclasses are listed below and are presented in an order from narrow-spectrum (penicillins) to broad-spectrum (carbapenem) β-lactam drugs.	Gram-negative bacteria have developed several pathways to β-lactam resistance. Perhaps the most concerning are β-lactamases, enzymes that destroy the β-lactam antibiotics. Some β-lactamases destroy narrow spectrum drugs (e.g., only active against penicillins) while newer β-lactamases (e.g. carbapenemases found in carbapenem-resistant Enterobacteriaceae or CRE) are active against all β-lactam antibiotics.
β-lactam subclass:		
Penicillin, aminopenicillins, and early generation cephalosporins	Among the first antibiotics developed for treatment of bacterial infections. In the absence of resistance, these drugs are active against a broad range of bacterial pathogens.	Resistance among gram-negative bacteria is widespread. These drugs are rarely recommended as treatment for serious gram-negative infections.
β-lactamase inhibitor combinations	These drugs are still active against gram-negative bacteria that have β-lactamases with limited activity for destroying β-lactam antibiotics.	These drugs are important for treatment of serious gram- negative infections but resistance is increasing. Bacteria that are resistant to extended-spectrum cephalosporins and carbapenems are usually resistant to these drugs as well. New β-lactamase inhibitor combination drugs in development have the potential to overcome some, but not all, of resistance from the most potent β-lactamases such as those found in CRE.
Extended-spectrum Cephalosporins	These drugs have been a cornerstone for treatment of serious gram-negative infections for the past 20 years.	Resistant gram-negative infections first emerged in healthcare settings but now are also spreading in the community. When resistance occurs, a carbapenem is the only remaining β-lactam agent.

Drug Class	Important Characteristics	Resistance and Other Limitations
Carbapenems	A broad-spectrum β-lactam antibiotic that is considered the last resort for treatment of serious gram-negative infections.	CRE infections are spreading in healthcare facilities throughout the United States and the world. It is reasonable to expect that this resistance will expand to bacteria that circulate in the community, as witnessed by extended-spectrum β-lactamase producing bacteria. Carbapenem resistance can also be found among other gram-negative bacteria including *Pseudomonas* and *Acinetobacter spp.* Once bacteria become resistant to carbapenems, they are usually resistant to all β-lactams.
Fluoroquinolones	These are broad-spectrum antibiotics that are often given orally, making them convenient to use in both inpatients and outpatients.	Resistant bacteria develop quickly with increased use in a patient population. Increased use is also associated with an increase in infections caused by fluoroquinolone-resistant, hyper-virulent strains of *Clostridium difficile*.
Aminoglycosides	These drugs are often used in combination with β-lactam drugs for the treatment of serious gram-negative infections.	Despite growing resistance problems, these drugs continue to be an important therapeutic option. However, clinicians rarely use these drugs alone because of concerns with resistance and side effects.
Tetracyclines & Glycyclines	Tetracyclines are not a first-line treatment option for serious gram negative infections; however, with increasing resistance to other drug classes, tetracyclines are considered as a treatment option. Glycyclines (i.e., tigecycline) are often considered for treatment of multidrug-resistant gram-negative infections.	Tigecycline is a drug that does not distribute evenly in the body, so it is often used in combination with other drugs depending upon the site of infection. Resistance to tigecycline has emerged but it is still relatively uncommon.
Polymyxins	These drugs are an older class that fell out of favor because of toxicity concerns. Now they are often used as a "last resort" agent for treatment of multidrug-resistant gram-negative infections.	Because these are generic drugs, there are limited contemporary data on proper dosing. In addition, resistance is emerging, but there are limited data guiding the accurate detection of resistance in hospital labs. As a result, use of these drugs present significant challenges for clinicians. In the absence of a drug sponsor, FDA and NIH are funding studies to fill these critical information gaps.

People at Especially High Risk

As antibiotic resistance grows, the antibiotics used to treat infections do not work as well or at all. The loss of effective antibiotic treatments will not only cripple the ability to fight routine infectious diseases but will also undermine treatment of infectious complications in patients with other diseases. Many of the advances in medical treatment—joint replacements, organ transplants, cancer therapy, and treatment of chronic diseases such as diabetes, asthma, rheumatoid arthritis—are dependent on the ability to fight infections with antibiotics. If that ability is lost, the ability to safely offer people many life-saving and life-improving modern medical advantages will be lost with it. For example:

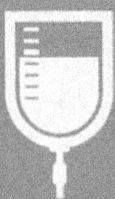

CANCER CHEMOTHERAPY

People receiving chemotherapy are often at risk for developing an infection when their white blood cell count is low. For these patients, any infection can quickly become serious and effective antibiotics are critical for protecting the patient from severe complications or death.

COMPLEX SURGERY

Patients who receive cardiac bypass, joint replacements, and other complex surgeries are at risk of a surgical site infection (SSI). These infections can make recovery from surgery more difficult because they can cause additional illness, stress, cost, and even death. For some, but not all surgeries, antibiotics are given before surgery to help prevent infections.

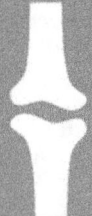

RHEUMATOID ARTHRITIS

Inflammatory arthritis affects the immune system, which controls how well the body fights off infections. People with certain types of arthritis have a higher risk of getting infections. Also, many medications given to treat inflammatory arthritis can weaken the immune system. Effective antibiotics help ensure that arthritis patients can continue to receive treatment.

DIALYSIS FOR END-STAGE RENAL DISEASE

Patients who undergo dialysis treatment have an increased risk for getting a bloodstream infection. In fact, bloodstream infections are the second leading cause of death in dialysis patients. Infections also complicate heart disease, the leading cause of death in diaysis patients. Infection risk is higher in these patients because they have weakened immune systems and often require catheters or needles to enter their bloodstream. Effective antibiotics help ensure that dialysis patients can continue to receive life-saving treatment.

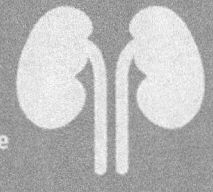

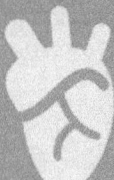

ORGAN AND BONE MARROW TRANSPLANTS

Transplant recipients are more vulnerable to infections. Because a patient undergoes complex surgery and receives medicine to weaken the immune system for a year or more, the risk of infection is high. It is estimated that 1% of organs transplanted in the United States each year carry a disease that comes from the donor—either an infection or cancer. Effective antibiotics help ensure that organ transplants remain possible.

Antibiotics are responsible for almost 1 out of 5 emergency department visits for adverse drug events. Antibiotics are the most common cause of emergency department visits for adverse drug events in children under 18 years of age.

- Antibiotics are powerful drugs that are generally safe and very helpful in fighting disease, but there are times when antibiotics can actually be harmful.

- Antibiotics can have side effects, including allergic reactions and a potentially deadly diarrhea caused by the bacteria *Clostridium difficile (C. difficile)*. Antibiotics can also interfere with the action of other drugs a patient may be taking for another condition. These unintended reactions to antibiotics are called adverse drug events.

- When someone takes an antibiotic that they do not need, they are needlessly exposed to the side effects of the drug and do not get any benefit from it.

- Moreover, taking an antibiotic when it is not needed can lead to the development of antibiotic resistance. When resistance develops, antibiotics may not be able to stop future infections. Every time someone takes an antibiotic they don't need, they increase their risk of developing a resistant infection in the future.

Types of Adverse Drug Events Related to Antibiotics

Allergic Reactions

Every year, there are more than 140,000 emergency department visits for reactions to antibiotics. Almost four out of five (79%) emergency department visits for antibiotic-related adverse drug events are due to an allergic reaction. These reactions can range from mild rashes and itching to serious blistering skin reactions swelling of the face and throat, and breathing problems. Minimizing unnecessary antibiotic use is the best way to reduce the risk of adverse drug events from antibiotics. Patients should tell their doctors about any past drug reactions or allergies.

C. difficile

C. difficile causes diarrhea linked to at least 14,000 American deaths each year. When a person takes antibiotics, good bacteria that protect against infection are destroyed for several months. During this time, patients can get sick from *C. difficile* picked up from contaminated surfaces or spread from a healthcare provider's hands. Those most at risk are people, especially older adults, who take antibiotics and also get medical care. Take antibiotics exactly and only as prescribed.

Drug Interactions and Side Effects

Antibiotics can interact with other drugs patients take, making those drugs or the antibiotics less effective. Some drug combinations can worsen the side effects of the antibiotic or other drug. Common side effects of antibiotics include nausea, diarrhea, and stomach pain. Sometimes these symptoms can lead to dehydration and other problems. Patients should ask their doctors about drug interactions and the potential side effects of antibiotics. The doctor should be told immediately if a patient has any side effects from antibiotics.

GAPS IN KNOWLEDGE
OF ANTIBIOTIC RESISTANCE

LIMITED NATIONAL, STATE, AND FEDERAL CAPACITY TO DETECT AND RESPOND TO URGENT AND EMERGING ANTIBIOTIC RESISTANCE THREATS

Even for critical pathogens of concern like carbapenem-resistant Enterobacteriaceae (CRE) and *Neisseria gonorrhoeae*, we do not have a complete picture of the domestic incidence, prevalence, mortality, and cost of resistance.

CURRENTLY, THERE IS NO SYSTEMATIC INTERNATIONAL SURVEILLANCE OF ANTIBIOTIC RESISTANCE THREATS

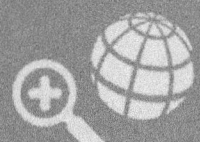

Today, the international identification of antibiotic resistance threats occurs through domestic importation of novel antibiotic resistance threats or through identification of overseas outbreaks.

DATA ON ANTIBIOTIC USE IN HUMAN HEALTHCARE AND IN AGRICULTURE ARE NOT SYSTEMATICALLY COLLECTED

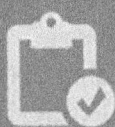

Routine systems of reporting and benchmarking antibiotic use wherever it occurs need to be piloted and scaled nationwide.

PROGRAMS TO IMPROVE ANTIBIOTIC PRESCRIBING ARE NOT WIDELY USED IN THE UNITED STATES

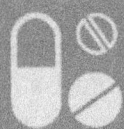

These inpatient and outpatient programs hold great promise for reducing antibiotic resistance threats, improving patient outcomes, and saving healthcare dollars.

ADVANCED TECHNOLOGIES CAN IDENTIFY THREATS MUCH FASTER THAN CURRENT PRACTICE

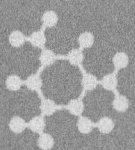

Advanced molecular detection (AMD) technologies, which can identify AR threats much faster than current practice, are not being used as widely as necessary in the United States.

Developing Resistance

Timeline of Key Antibiotic Resistance Events

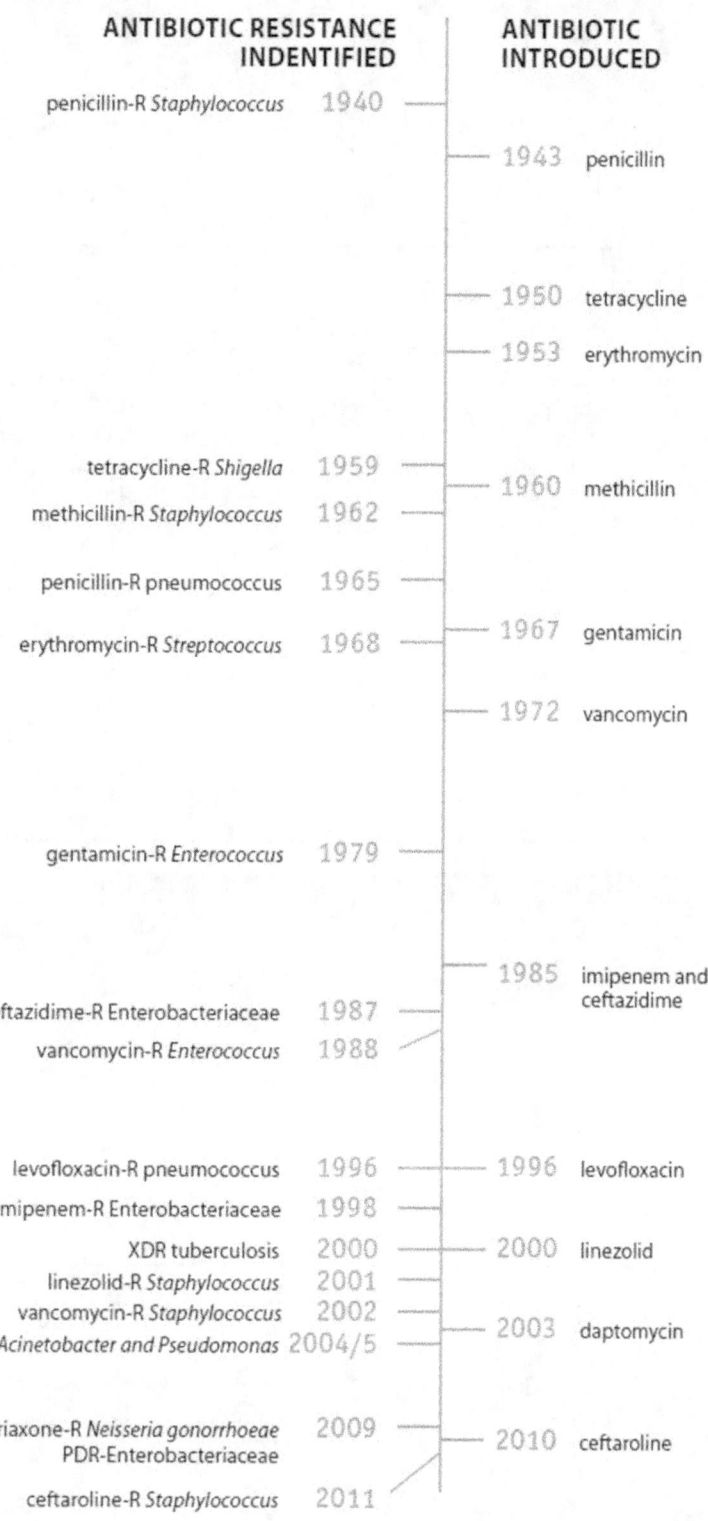

Dates are based upon early reports of resistance in the literature. In the case of pan drug-resistant (PDR)- *Acinetobacter* and *Pseudomonas*, the date is based upon reports of healthcare transmission or outbreaks. Note: penicillin was in limited use prior to widespread population usage in 1943.

ANTIBIOTIC RESISTANCE INDENTIFIED		ANTIBIOTIC INTRODUCED	
penicillin-R *Staphylococcus*	1940		
		1943	penicillin
		1950	tetracycline
		1953	erythromycin
tetracycline-R *Shigella*	1959	1960	methicillin
methicillin-R *Staphylococcus*	1962		
penicillin-R pneumococcus	1965		
erythromycin-R *Streptococcus*	1968	1967	gentamicin
		1972	vancomycin
gentamicin-R *Enterococcus*	1979		
		1985	imipenem and ceftazidime
ceftazidime-R Enterobacteriaceae	1987		
vancomycin-R *Enterococcus*	1988		
levofloxacin-R pneumococcus	1996	1996	levofloxacin
imipenem-R Enterobacteriaceae	1998		
XDR tuberculosis	2000	2000	linezolid
linezolid-R *Staphylococcus*	2001		
vancomycin-R *Staphylococcus*	2002	2003	daptomycin
PDR-*Acinetobacter and Pseudomonas*	2004/5		
ceftriaxone-R *Neisseria gonorrhoeae* PDR-Enterobacteriaceae	2009	2010	ceftaroline
ceftaroline-R *Staphylococcus*	2011		

FIGHTING BACK AGAINST ANTIBIOTIC RESISTANCE

Four Core Actions to Prevent Antibiotic Resistance

1 PREVENTING INFECTIONS, PREVENTING THE SPREAD OF RESISTANCE

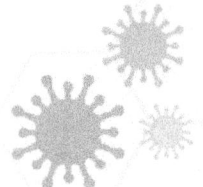

Avoiding infections in the first place reduces the amount of antibiotics that have to be used and reduces the likelihood that resistance will develop during therapy. There are many ways that drug-resistant infections can be prevented: immunization, safe food preparation, handwashing, and using antibiotics as directed and only when necessary. In addition, preventing infections also prevents the spread of resistant bacteria.

2 TRACKING

CDC gathers data on antibiotic-resistant infections, causes of infections and whether there are particular reasons (risk factors) that caused some people to get a resistant infection. With that information, experts can develop specific strategies to prevent those infections and prevent the resistant bacteria from spreading.

3 IMPROVING ANTIBIOTIC PRESCRIBING/STEWARDSHIP

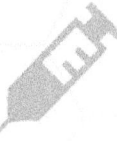
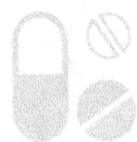

Perhaps the single most important action needed to greatly slow down the development and spread of antibiotic-resistant infections is to change the way antibiotics are used. Up to half of antibiotic use in humans and much of antibiotic use in animals is unnecessary and inappropriate and makes everyone less safe. Stopping even some of the inappropriate and unnecessary use of antibiotics in people and animals would help greatly in slowing down the spread of resistant bacteria. This commitment to always use antibiotics appropriately and safely—only when they are needed to treat disease, and to choose the right antibiotics and to administer them in the right way in every case—is known as antibiotic stewardship.

4 DEVELOPING NEW DRUGS AND DIAGNOSTIC TESTS

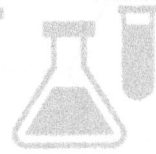

Because antibiotic resistance occurs as part of a natural process in which bacteria evolve, it can be slowed but not stopped. Therefore, we will always need new antibiotics to keep up with resistant bacteria as well as new diagnostic tests to track the development of resistance.

1. PREVENTING INFECTIONS, PREVENTING THE SPREAD OF RESISTANCE

Preventing infections from developing reduces the amount of antibiotics used. This reduction in antibiotic use, in turn, slows the pace of antibiotic resistance. Preventing infections also prevents the spread of resistant bacteria. Antibiotic-resistant infections can be prevented in many ways. This section focuses on CDC's works to prevent antibiotic-resistant infections in healthcare settings, in the community, and in food.

CDC's Work to Prevent Antibiotic Resistance in the Community

Antibiotic-resistant infections outside of the hospital setting were rare until recently. Today, resistant infections that can be transmitted in the community include tuberculosis and respiratory infections caused by *Streptococcus pneumoniae*, skin infections caused by methicillin-resistant *Staphylococcus aureus,* and sexually transmitted infections such as gonorrhea.

CDC works to prevent antibiotic resistance in the community by providing systems to track infections and changes in resistance; improving prescribing at national, regional, and local levels; and limiting or interrupting the spread of infections. These activities are similar to the strategies used in medical settings, but the approach can differ because the population (potentially everyone) is large and the settings are different. Here are some examples of the strategies CDC uses to prevent antibiotic resistance in communities:

Tracking Community Infections and Resistance

These programs are examples of CDC's effort to identify critical infections in the community and monitor resistance trends.

- **Active Bacterial Core surveillance (ABCs):** Tracking infections caused by *Neisseria meningitidis, Streptococcus pneumoniae,* Groups A and B *Streptococcus,* and methicillin-resistant *Staphylococcus aureus*

- **Gonococcal Isolate Surveillance Project (GISP):** Collecting isolates from gonorrhea infections to monitor antibiotic resistance

- **National Tuberculosis Surveillance System (NTSS):** National Electronic Disease Surveillance System (NEDSS)-based reporting of tuberculosis cases including resistance data

- **Healthcare-Associated Infections-Community Interface (HAIC):** Tracking infections with *C. difficile* and with multidrug-resistant gram-negative microorganisms.

Improving Antibiotic Prescribing

Prescribing antibiotics when they are not needed or prescribing the wrong antibiotic in outpatient settings such as doctors' offices is common. In some cases, doctors might not order laboratory tests to confirm that bacteria are causing the infection, and therefore the antibiotic might be unnecessarily prescribed. In other cases, patients demand treatment for conditions such as a cold when antibiotics are not needed and will not help. Likewise, healthcare providers can be too willing to satisfy a patient's expectation for an antibiotic prescription. CDC manages the Get Smart program, a national campaign to improve antibiotic prescribing and use in both outpatient and inpatient settings, and supports a variety of state-based programs modeled on the national effort. CDC provides local public health authorities with messages and resources for improving antibiotic use in outpatient settings and is now working with a variety of partners to identify new approaches for improving antibiotic use.

Limiting and Interrupting the Spread of Antibiotic-Resistant Infections in the Community

Preventing the spread of infection in the community is a significant challenge, and many prevention interventions are used, depending on the type of infection and the route of transmission.

Here are some examples of CDC's activities to limit and interrupt the spread of antibiotic-resistant community infections:

- Contact Tracing: A prevention strategy that has proven successful is tracking cases (individuals who are infected) and tracing contacts (people who have had contact with a case that puts them at risk for infection as well).This process is used to ensure that all persons requiring an intervention such as treatment, prophylaxis, or temporary isolation from the general public are identified and managed appropriately. This approach is resource intensive, but it has successfully limited transmission of infections including tuberculosis, gonorrhea, and meningococcus.

- Vaccination: There are few vaccines for antibiotic-resistant bacteria, but the *S. pneumoniae* vaccine has proven that an effective vaccine can reduce antibiotic resistance rates. The vaccine targets certain types of the bacteria, even if it is a resistant type, and reduces the overall number of infections, including those that are caused by resistant strains. The first version of the vaccine was introduced in 2000 and reduced the frequency of antibiotic-resistant infections, but it did not protect against a particular strain of *S. pneumoniae* called serotype 19A.This strain became increasingly resistant to antibiotics and caused more infections because the vaccine did not offer protection. A new version of the vaccine,

128

approved for use in 2010, protects against serotype 19A.As a result, the rate of resistant pneumococcal infections is decreasing.

- Treatment Guidelines: The spread of antibiotic resistance can be prevented if infections are effectively treated before the pathogen is spread to others. For some infections, laboratory tests for guiding treatment are not easily available or the turn-around time is slow or incomplete. This is the case for treating gonorrhea and tuberculosis. For these infections, healthcare providers rely on treatment guidelines for proper management of infections.CDC monitors resistance trends in *Neisseria gonorrhoeae* (the cause of gonorrhea) and *Mycobacterium tuberculosis* (the cause of tuberculosis) and publishes treatment guidelines to limit the progression of these diseases and the spread of bacteria.

- Promotion of Safe Sex: Increases in the spread of drug-resistant *Neisseria gonorrhoeae* poses unique challenges. To prevent transmission of this infection, CDC works to promote safer sexual behaviors such as abstinence, mutual monogamy, and correct and consistent condom use.

Preventing Infections: CDC's Work to Prevent Antibiotic Resistance in Food

Each year, millions of people in the United States become sick from foodborne and other enteric (gastrointestinal) infections. While many of these infections are mild and do not require treatment, antibiotics can be lifesaving in severe infections. Antibiotic resistance compromises our ability to treat these infections and is a serious threat to public health. Preventing resistant enteric infections requires a multifaceted approach and partnerships because bacteria that cause some infections, such as salmonellosis and campylobacteriosis, have animal reservoirs, while other bacteria, such as those that cause shigellosis and typhoid fever, have human reservoirs. To prevent antibiotic-resistant foodborne infections, CDC works closely with state and local health departments; with the U.S. Food and Drug Administration (FDA), which regulates antibiotics, many foods, animal feed, and other products; and with the U.S. Department of Agriculture (USDA), which regulates meat, poultry, and egg products.

Tracking Antibiotic Resistance

In 1996, the National Antimicrobial Resistance Monitoring System (NARMS) was established as a collaboration among CDC, FDA, USDA, and state and local public health departments. This national public health surveillance system tracks antibiotic resistance among *Salmonella, Campylobacter,* and other bacteria transmitted commonly through food. NARMS tests bacteria from humans (CDC), retail meats (FDA), and food-producing animals (USDA) in the United States. The primary objectives of the NARMS program are to:

129

- Monitor trends in antibiotic resistance among enteric bacteria from humans, retail meats, and food-producing animals.

- Disseminate information on antibiotic resistance to promote interventions that reduce antibiotic resistance among foodborne bacteria.

- Conduct research to better understand the emergence, persistence, and spread of antibiotic resistance.

- Provide data that assist the FDA in making decisions about approving safe and effective antibiotic drugs for animals.

The CDC reference laboratory conducts antibiotic susceptibility testing on isolates from sporadic cases and outbreaks of illness. The lab also confirms and studies bacteria that have new antibiotic resistance patterns. NARMS provides information about patterns of emerging resistance among enteric pathogens to stakeholders, including federal regulatory agencies, policymakers, consumer advocacy groups, industry, and the public, to guide public health prevention and policy efforts that protect people from resistant infections. For more information about NARMS: www.cdc.gov/narms.

Improving Antibiotic Use

Antibiotics are widely used in food-producing animals, and according to data published by FDA, there are more kilograms of antibiotics sold in the United States for food-producing animals than for people.(http://www.fda.gov/downloads/ForIndustry/UserFees/ AnimalDrugUserFeeActADUFA/UCM338170.pdf).This use contributes to the emergence of antibiotic-resistant bacteria in food-producing animals. Resistant bacteria in food-producing animals are of particular concern because these animals serve as carriers. Resistant bacteria can contaminate the foods that come from those animals, and people who consume these foods can develop antibiotic-resistant infections. Antibiotics must be used judiciously in humans and animals because both uses contribute to not only the emergence, but also the persistence and spread of antibiotic-resistant bacteria.

Scientists around the world have provided strong evidence that antibiotic use in food-producing animals can harm public health through the following sequence of events:

- Use of antibiotics in food-producing animals allows antibiotic-resistant bacteria to thrive while susceptible bacteria are suppressed or die.

130

- Resistant bacteria can be transmitted from food-producing animals to humans through the food supply.

- Resistant bacteria can cause infections in humans.

- Infections caused by resistant bacteria can result in adverse health consequences for humans.

Because of the link between antibiotic use in food-producing animals and the occurrence of antibiotic-resistant infections in humans, antibiotics should be used in food-producing animals only under veterinary oversight and only to manage and treat infectious diseases, not to promote growth.CDC encourages and supports efforts to minimize inappropriate use of antibiotics in humans and animals, including FDA's strategy to promote the judicious use of antibiotics that are important in treating humans (http://www.fda.gov/ AnimalVeterinary/SafetyHealth/AntimicrobialResistance/JudiciousUseofAntimicrobial s/ default.htm).CDC supports FDA's plan to implement draft guidance in 2013 that will operationalize this strategy (http://www.fda.gov/downloads/AnimalVeterinary/ GuidanceComplianceEnforcement/GuidanceforIndustry/UCM299624.pdf).CDC has also contributed to a training curriculum for veterinarians on prudent antibiotic use in animals. CDC's efforts to improve antibiotic prescribing in humans are described in other sections of this report.

Preventing Infections

Efforts to prevent foodborne and other enteric infections help to reduce both antibiotic-resistant infections and antibiotic-susceptible infections (those that can be treated effectively with antibiotics).CDC activities that help prevent these infections include:

- Estimating how much foodborne illness occurs.

- Monitoring trends in foodborne infections.

- Investigating outbreaks and sporadic cases of foodborne illness to stop outbreaks and improve prevention.

- Attributing illnesses to specific foods and settings.

- Tracking and responding to changes in resistance.

- Determining the sources of antibiotic-resistant enteric infections.

- Educating consumers and food workers about safe food handling practices.

- Identifying and educating groups at high risk for infection.

- Promoting proper handwashing.

- Strengthening the capacity of state and local health departments to detect, respond to, and report foodborne infections.

- Developing better diagnostic tools to rapidly and accurately find sources of contamination.

Providing recommendations for travelers on safe food and clean water.

2. TRACKING RESISTANCE PATTERNS

CDC gathers data on antibiotic-resistant infections, causes of infections, and whether there are particular reasons (risk factors) that caused some people to get a resistant infection. With that information, experts develop specific strategies to prevent those infections and prevent the resistant bacteria from spreading.

CDC's Antibiotic Resistance and Antibiotic-Resistant Infections Tracking Platform

Tracking Networks	Data Collected	Resistant Bacteria/Fungus[3]

EIP
 	
Emerging Infections Program
 	
There are three main programs within the EIP:
 	
    ABCs: Active Bacterial Core surveillance
 	
    HAIC: Healthcare-Associated Infections-Community Interface
 	
    FoodNet: Foodborne Diseases Active Surveillance Network
	A network of public health-academic-hospital collaborations in 10 states. It provides access to bacterial and fungal samples for testing and detailed clinical case data.
	
	The three main programs within EIP collect different types of resistance data:
	
	    ABCs provides clinical information and resistance data for bacteria that cause infections predominately in the community.
	
	    The HAIC provides clinical information and resistance data for bacteria and fungi that cause infections at the intersection of healthcare and the general community.
	
	    FoodNet supplies clinical and epidemiologic data on some human isolates in the National Antimicrobial Resistance Monitoring System (NARMS).
		ABCs:
		
		Streptococcus pneumoniae
		
		Groups A and B *Streptococcus*
		
		Methicillin-resistant *Staphylococcus aureus*
		
		HAIC:
		
		C. difficile
		
		Candida (a fungus)
		
		Carbapenem-R Enterobacteriaceae
		
		MDR *Acinetobacter*
		
		FoodNet: (see NARMS list)

NARMS National Antimicrobial Resistance Monitoring System	A national public health surveillance system that tracks changes in the susceptibility of foodborne and other enteric bacteria to antibiotics of human and veterinary medical importance. NARMS is a collaboration among CDC, FDA, USDA, and state and local health departments. CDC tests bacterial isolates from humans, while FDA and USDA test isolates from retail meats and food animals.	*Salmonella* *Campylobacter* *Shigella*

Tracking Networks	Data Collected	Resistant Bacteria/Fungus[3]
NHSN National Healthcare Safety Network	A system that collects and provides data on infections and drug-resistance in healthcare settings. Since NHSN collects data directly from healthcare facilities, it can provide facility-level information on healthcare-associated infections and antibiotic resistance (and in the future, on antibiotic use).	*Staphylococcus aureus* *Enterococcus* Enterobacteriaceae *Acinetobacter* *Pseudomonas aeruginosa* *Candida* (a fungus)
GISP Gonococcal Isolate Surveillance Program	A program to track antibiotic resistance data for gonococcal isolates. Isolates are collected from sexually transmitted disease clinics in approximately 28 cities.	*Neisseria gonorrhoeae*
NTSS National Tuberculosis Surveillance System	National Electronic Disease Surveillance System (NEDSS)-based reporting of tuberculosis cases including resistance data. Public health departments from 50 states and the US territories contribute data.	*Mycobacterium tuberculosis*

[3]ABCs also includes surveillance for *Neisseria meningitidis* and *Haemophilus influenzae*. NARMS also includes surveillance for *E. coli O157* and *Vibrio* (non-*V. cholerae*).

3. ANTIBIOTIC STEWARDSHIP: IMPROVING PRESCRIBING AND USE

Antibiotics were first used to treat serious infections in the 1940s. Since then, antibiotics have saved millions of lives and transformed modern medicine. During the last 70 years, however, bacteria have shown the ability to become resistant to every antibiotic that has been developed. And the more antibiotics are used, the more quickly bacteria develop resistance *(see the Antibiotic Resistance Timeline in this report)*.

Anytime antibiotics are used, this puts biological pressure on bacteria that promotes the development of resistance. When antibiotics are needed to prevent or treat disease, they should always be used. But research has shown that as much as 50% of the time, antibiotics are prescribed when they are not needed or they are misused (for example, a patient is given the wrong dose). This not only fails to help patients; it might cause harm. Like every other drug, antibiotics have side effects and can also interact or interfere with the effects of other medicines. This inappropriate use of antibiotics unnecessarily promotes antibiotic resistance.

Antibiotics are a limited resource. The more that antibiotics are used today, the less likely they will still be effective in the future. Therefore, doctors and other health professionals around the world are increasingly adopting the principles of responsible antibiotic use, often called antibiotic stewardship. Stewardship is a commitment to always use antibiotics only when they are necessary to treat, and in some cases prevent, disease; to choose the right antibiotics; and to administer them in the right way in every case. Effective stewardship ensures that every patient gets the maximum benefit from the antibiotics, avoids unnecessary harm from allergic reactions and side effects, and helps preserve the life-saving potential of these drugs for the future. Efforts to improve the responsible use of antibiotics have not only demonstrated these benefits but have also been shown to improve outcomes and save healthcare facilities money in pharmacy costs.

Antibiotic Prescriptions per 1000 Persons of All Ages According to State, 2010

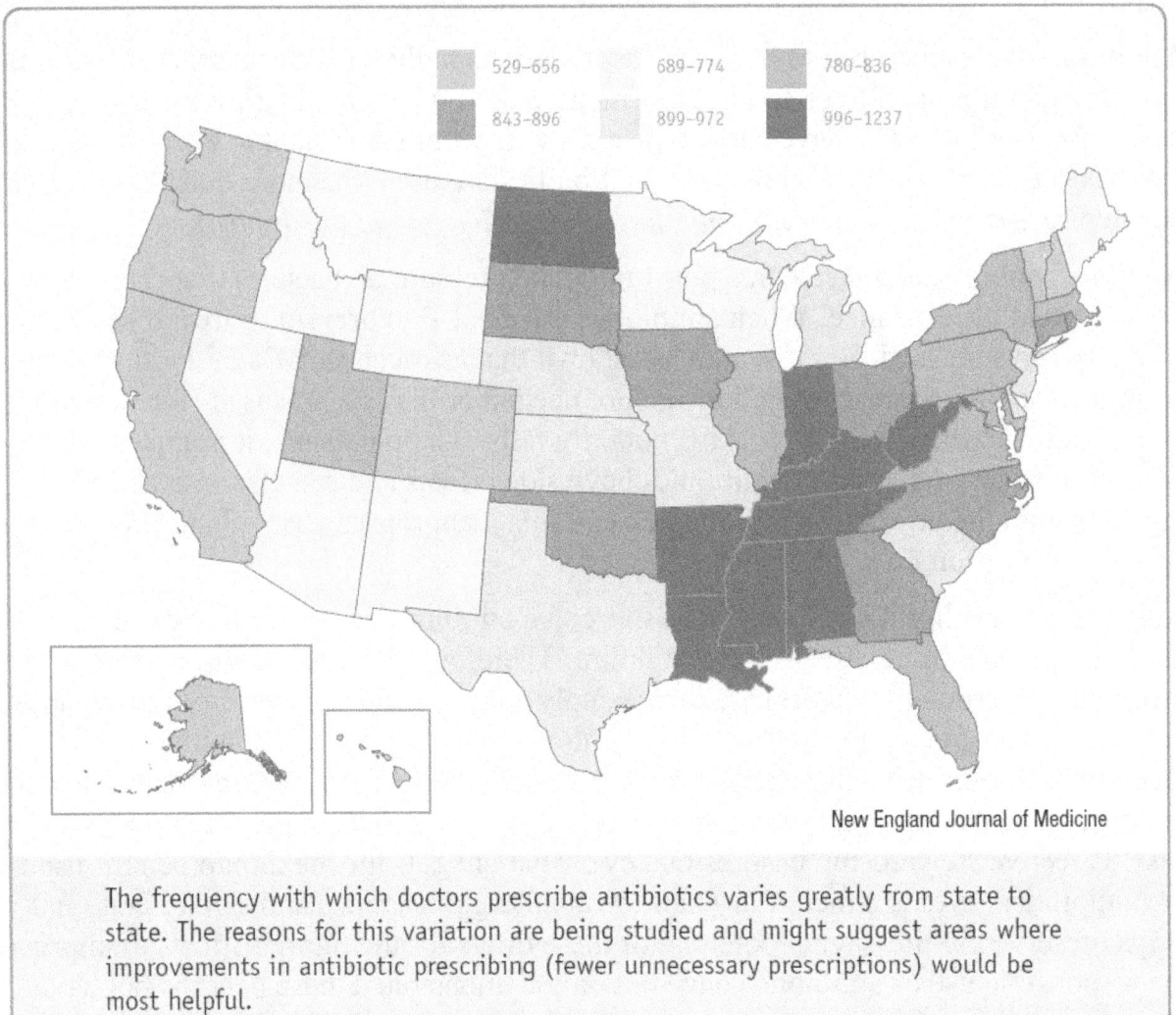

529–656	689–774	780–836
843–896	899–972	996–1237

New England Journal of Medicine

The frequency with which doctors prescribe antibiotics varies greatly from state to state. The reasons for this variation are being studied and might suggest areas where improvements in antibiotic prescribing (fewer unnecessary prescriptions) would be most helpful.

ANTIBIOTIC STEWARDSHIP

IN YOUR FACILITY WILL

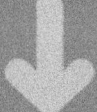 **DECREASE**

- ANTIBIOTIC RESISTANCE
- C. DIFFICILE INFECTIONS
- COSTS

INCREASE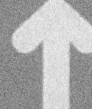

- GOOD PATIENT OUTCOMES

PROMOTE ANTIBIOTIC BEST PRACTICES— A FIRST STEP IN ANTIBIOTIC STEWARDSHIP

- ENSURE ALL ORDERS HAVE DOSE, DURATION, AND INDICATIONS
- GET CULTURES BEFORE STARTING ANTIBIOTICS
- TAKE AN "ANTIBIOTIC TIMEOUT" REASSESSING ANTIBIOTICS AFTER 48–72 HOURS

ANTIBIOTIC STEWARDSHIP PROGRAMS ARE A "WIN-WIN" FOR ALL INVOLVED

A UNIVERSITY OF MARYLAND STUDY SHOWED ONE ANTIBIOTIC STEWARDSHIP PROGRAM **SAVED A TOTAL OF $17 MILLION** OVER EIGHT YEARS

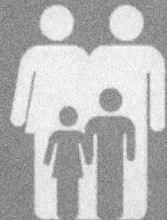

ANTIBIOTIC STEWARDSHIP HELPS **IMPROVE PATIENT CARE AND SHORTEN HOSPTIAL STAYS,** THUS **BENEFITING PATIENTS AS WELL AS HOSPITALS**

4. DEVELOPING NEW ANTIBIOTICS AND DIAGNOSTIC TESTS

Because antibiotic resistance occurs as part of a natural evolution process, it can be significantly slowed but not stopped. Therefore, new antibiotics will always be needed to keep up with resistant bacteria as well as new diagnostic tests to track the development of resistance.

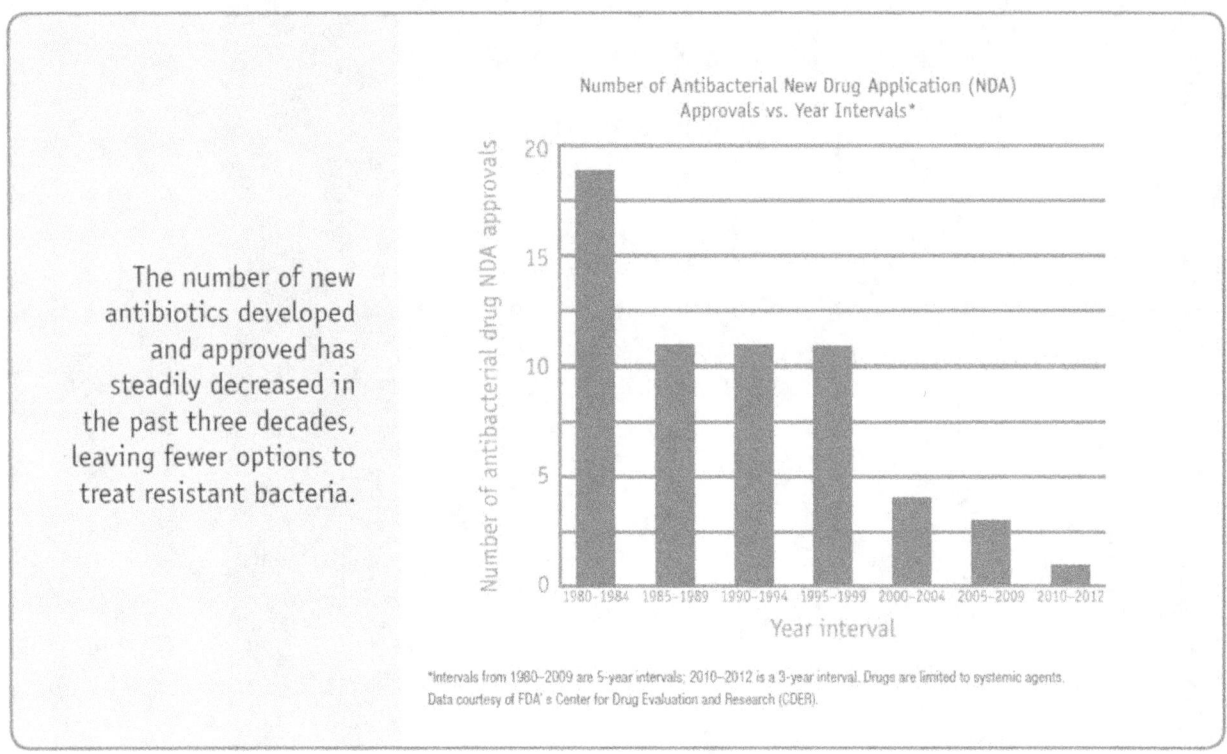

The number of new antibiotics developed and approved has steadily decreased in the past three decades, leaving fewer options to treat resistant bacteria.

*Intervals from 1980–2009 are 5-year intervals; 2010–2012 is a 3-year interval. Drugs are limited to systemic agents.
Data courtesy of FDA's Center for Drug Evaluation and Research (CDER).

Examples of Recently Approved Drugs

Drug Name	Year Approved	Key Targeted Pathogens	Drug's Use and Resistance Trends
Quinupristin/ Dalfoprisitin	1999	*Staphylococcus* *Streptococcus*	This is a combination of two drugs that can be used to treat gram-positive infections. Because side effects are common, this drug is usually not a first choice for therapy. Resistance in target pathogens has been described, but the percentage in the United States is still low.
Moxifloxacin	1999	Enterobacteriaceae *Staphylococcus* *Streptococcus*	Moxifloxacin, like other fluoroquinolones, demonstrates broad spectrum activity, and it can be used to treat a range of infections. Unfortunately, there is cross-resistance among the fluoroquinolones, and resistance is increasing in all targeted pathogens, especially Enterobacteriaceae.
Linezolid	2000	*Staphylococcus* *Enterococcus*	Linezolid can be used to treat serious gram-positive infections. Resistance has occurred but it is still uncommon.
Ertapenem	2001	Enterobacteriaceae *Staphylococcus* *Streptococcus*	Ertapenem is a carbapenem that can be used to treat a wide range of infections. Dissemination of carbapenem-resistant Enterobacteriaceae (CRE) is impacting the drug's overall effectiveness.
Gemifloxacin	2003	Enterobacteriaceae *Streptococcus*	Gemifloxacin is a fluoroquinolone that can be used to treat mild to moderate community-associated respiratory disease. Like moxifloxacin, there is cross-resistance with other fluoroquinolone drugs so resistance is increasing.
Daptomycin	2003	*Staphylococcus* *Streptococcus* *Enterococcus*	Daptomycin is often used for treatment of serious gram-positive infections. Resistance is emerging in all of the targeted pathogens, but the resistance rates are currently low.
Tigecycline	2005	Enterobacteriaceae *Staphylococcus* *Streptococcus* *Enterococcus*	Tigecycline is often one of the only active agents for carbapenem-resistant gram-negative infections, and resistance is emerging. However, even in the absence of resistance, the effectiveness of this agent for treatment of the most serious infections is a concern.
Doripenem	2007	Enterobacteriaceae *Pseudomonas aeruginosa* *Acinetobacter spp.* *Streptococcus spp.*	Doripenem is a carbapenem drug most commonly used to treat serious gram-negative infections. Dissemination of carbapenem-resistant gram-negative pathogens like CRE is reducing the overall effectiveness of this drug.
Telavancin	2008	*Staphylococcus* *Streptococcus* *Enterococcus*	Telavancin is approved for treatment of gram-positive skin and soft tissue infections. Use is limited because it is administered intravenously and is therefore difficult to use in an outpatient setting. In addition, it should not be used in a woman of childbearing age without a pregnancy test.

CURRENT ANTIBIOTIC RESISTANCE THREATS IN THE UNITED STATES, BY MICROORGANISM

This section includes summaries for each microorganism, grouped by threat level: URGENT, SERIOUS, and CONCERNING.

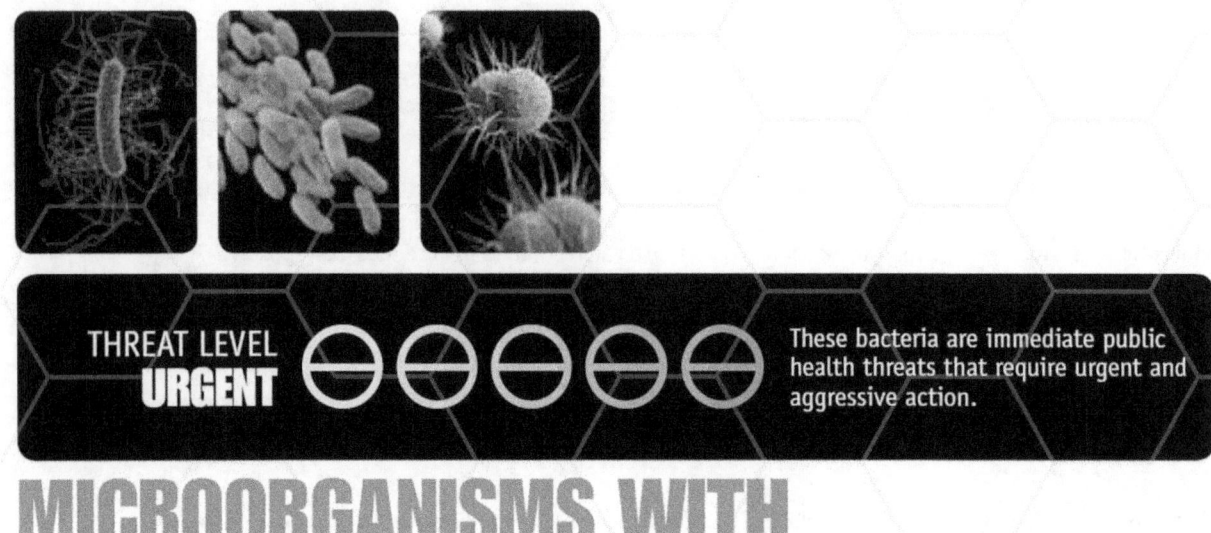

THREAT LEVEL
URGENT

These bacteria are immediate public health threats that require urgent and aggressive action.

MICROORGANISMS WITH A THREAT LEVEL OF URGENT

Clostridium difficile

Carbapenem-resistant **Enterobacteriaceae**

Drug-resistant *Neisseria gonorrhoeae*

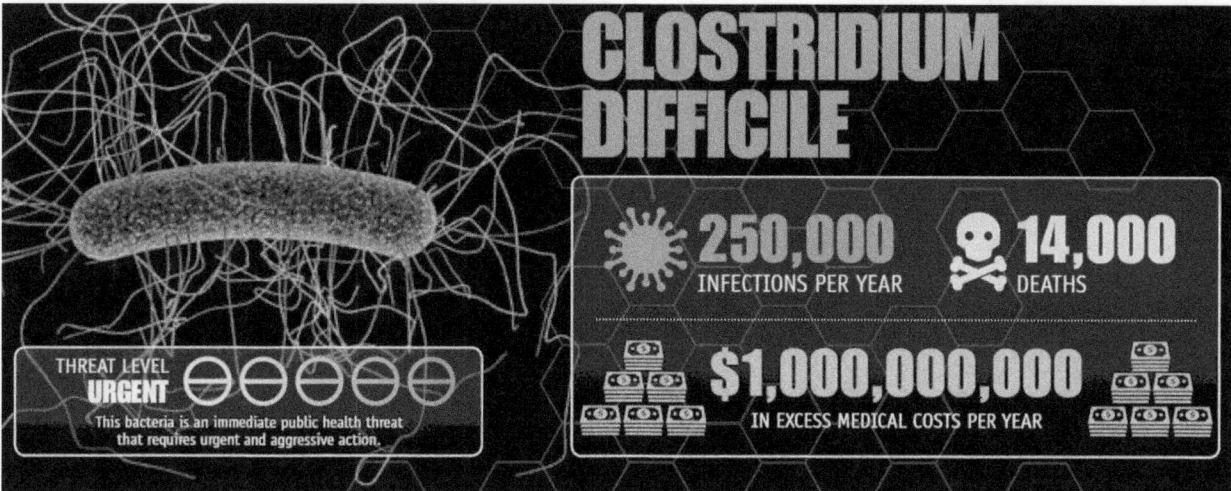

CLOSTRIDIUM DIFFICILE

250,000
INFECTIONS PER YEAR

14,000
DEATHS

$1,000,000,000
IN EXCESS MEDICAL COSTS PER YEAR

THREAT LEVEL
URGENT
This bacteria is an immediate public health threat
that requires urgent and aggressive action.

Clostridium difficile (C. difficile) causes life-threatening diarrhea. These infections mostly occur in people who have had both recent medical care and antibiotics. Often, *C. difficile* infections occur in hospitalized or recently hospitalized patients.

RESISTANCE OF CONCERN

- Although resistance to the antibiotics used to treat *C. difficile* infections is not yet a problem, the bacteria spreads rapidly because it is naturally resistant to many drugs used to treat other infections.

- In 2000, a stronger strain of the bacteria emerged. This strain is resistant to fluoroquinolone antibiotics, which are commonly used to treat other infections.

- This strain has spread throughout North America and Europe, infecting and killing more people wherever it spreads.

PUBLIC HEALTH THREAT

- 250,000 infections per year requiring hospitalization or affecting already hospitalized patients.

- 14,000 deaths per year.

- At least $1 billion in excess medical costs per year.

- Deaths related to *C. difficile* increased 400% between 2000 and 2007, in part because of a stronger bacteria strain that emerged.

- Almost half of infections occur in people younger than 65, but more than 90% of deaths occur in people 65 and older.

- About half of *C. difficile* infections first show symptoms in hospitalized or recently hospitalized patients, and half first show symptoms in nursing home patients or in people recently cared for in doctors' offices and clinics.

CLOSTRIDIUM DIFFICILE

FIGHTING THE SPREAD OF RESISTANCE

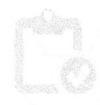

WHAT CDC IS DOING

- Tracking and reporting national progress toward preventing *C. difficile* infections.

- Promoting *C. difficile* prevention programs and providing gold-standard patient safety recommendations.

- Providing prevention expertise, as well as outbreak and laboratory assistance, to health departments and healthcare facilities.

WHAT YOU CAN DO

CEOs, Medical Officers, and other Healthcare Facility Leaders Can:

- Support better testing (nucleic acid amplification tests), tracking, and reporting of infections and prevention efforts.

- Ensure policies for rapid detection and isolation of patients with *C. difficile* are in place and followed.

- Assess hospital cleaning to be sure it is performed thoroughly, and augment this using an Environmental Protection Agency-approved, spore-killing disinfectant in rooms where *C. difficile* patients are treated.

- Notify other healthcare facilities about infectious diseases when patients transfer, especially between hospitals and nursing homes.

- Participate in a regional *C. difficile* prevention effort.

Healthcare Providers Can:

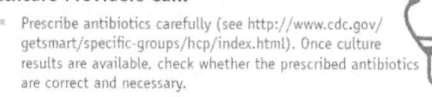

- Prescribe antibiotics carefully (see http://www.cdc.gov/getsmart/specific-groups/hcp/index.html). Once culture results are available, check whether the prescribed antibiotics are correct and necessary.

- Order a *C. difficile* test (preferably a nucleic acid amplification test) if the patient has had 3 or more unformed stools within 24 hours.

- Be aware of infection rates in your facility or practice, and follow infection control recommendations with every patient. This includes using contact precautions (gloves and gowns) and isolation for patients who are suspected to have *C. difficile*, and continuing those practices for those with positive test results.

Patients can:

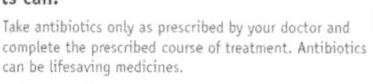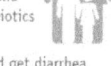

- Take antibiotics only as prescribed by your doctor and complete the prescribed course of treatment. Antibiotics can be lifesaving medicines.

- Tell your doctor if you have been on antibiotics and get diarrhea within a few months.

- Wash your hands before eating and after using the bathroom.

- Try to use a separate bathroom if you have diarrhea, or be sure the bathroom is cleaned well if someone with diarrhea has used it.

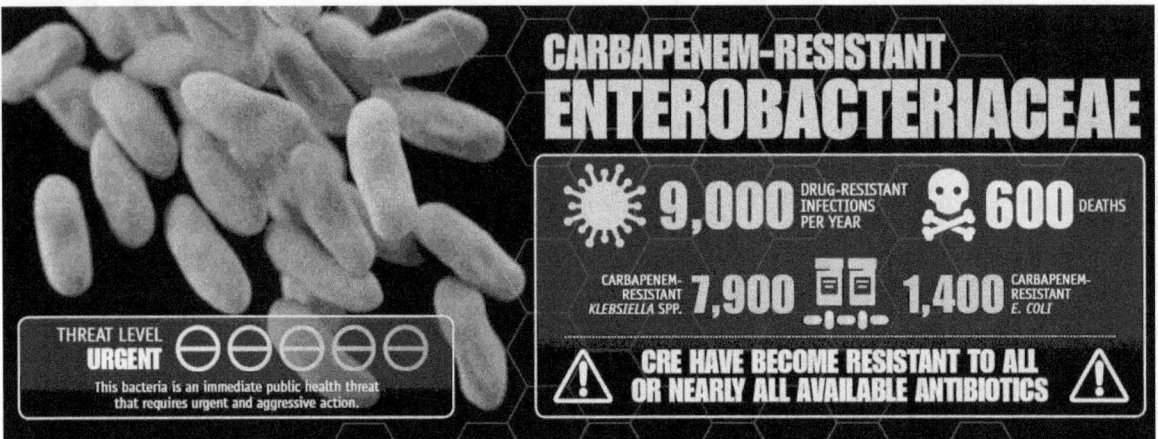

Untreatable and hard-to-treat infections from carbapenem-resistant Enterobacteriaceae (CRE) bacteria are on the rise among patients in medical facilities. CRE have become resistant to all or nearly all the antibiotics we have today. Almost half of hospital patients who get bloodstream infections from CRE bacteria die from the infection.

RESISTANCE OF CONCERN

- Some Enterobacteriaceae are resistant to nearly all antibiotics, including carbapenems, which are often considered the antibiotics of last resort.
- More than 9,000 healthcare-associated infections are caused by CRE each year.
- CDC laboratories have confirmed at least one type of CRE in healthcare facilities in 44 states.
- About 4% of U.S. short-stay hospitals had at least one patient with a serious CRE infection during the first half of 2012. About 18% of long-term acute care hospitals had one.

PUBLIC HEALTH THREAT

An estimated 140,000 healthcare-associated Enterobacteriaceae infections occur in the United States each year; about 9,300 of these are caused by CRE. Up to half of all bloodstream infections caused by CRE result in death. Fortunately, bloodstream infections account for a minority of all healthcare-associated infections caused by Enterobacteriaceae. Each year, approximately 600 deaths result from infections caused by the two most common types of CRE, carbapenem-resistant *Klebsiella* spp. and carbapenem-resistant *E. coli*.

	Percentage of Enterobacteriaceae healthcare-associated infections resistant to carbapenems	Estimated number of infections	Estimated number of deaths attributed
Carbapenem-Resistant *Klebsiella* spp.	11%	7,900	520
Carbapenem-resistant *E. coli*	2%	1,400	90

For more information about data methods and references, please see technical appendix.

142

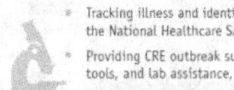

CARBAPENEM-RESISTANT ENTEROBACTERIACEAE

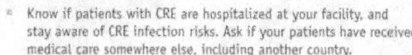

FIGHTING THE SPREAD OF RESISTANCE

WHAT CDC IS DOING

- Tracking illness and identifying risk factors for CRE infections using two systems, the National Healthcare Safety Network and the Emerging Infections Program.
- Providing CRE outbreak support, such as staff expertise, prevention guidelines, tools, and lab assistance, to states and facilities.
- Developing tests and prevention programs to identify and control CRE. CDC's "Detect and Protect" effort (http://www.cdc.gov/hai/pdfs/cre/CDC_DetectProtect.pdf) supports regional CRE programs.
- Helping medical facilities improve antibiotic prescribing practices.

WHAT YOU CAN DO

States and Communities Can:

- Know CRE trends in your region.
- Coordinate regional CRE tracking and control efforts in areas with CRE. Areas not yet or rarely affected by CRE infections can be proactive in CRE prevention efforts.
- Require facilities to alert each other when transferring patients with any infection.
- Consider including CRE infections on your state's Notifiable Diseases list.

Healthcare CEOs, Medical Officers, and Other Healthcare Facility Leaders Can:

- Require and strictly enforce CDC guidance for CRE detection, prevention, tracking, and reporting.
- Make sure your lab can accurately identify CRE and alert clinical and infection prevention staff when these bacteria are present.
- Know CRE trends in your facility and in the facilities around you.
- When transferring a patient, require staff to notify the other facility about infections, including CRE.
- Join or start regional CRE prevention efforts, and promote wise antibiotic use.

Health Care Providers Can:

- Know if patients with CRE are hospitalized at your facility, and stay aware of CRE infection risks. Ask if your patients have received medical care somewhere else, including another country.
- Follow infection control recommendations with every patient, using contact precautions for patients with CRE. Whenever possible, dedicate rooms, equipment, and staff to CRE patients.
- Prescribe antibiotics wisely (http://www.cdc.gov/getsmart/healthcare). Use culture results to modify prescriptions if needed.
- Remove temporary medical devices as soon as possible.

Patients Can:

- Tell your doctor if you have been hospitalized in another facility or country.
- Take antibiotics only as prescribed.
- Insist that everyone wash their hands before touching you.

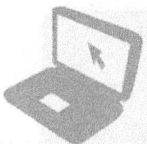

ONLINE RESOURCES

Vital Signs, March 2013: Making Health Care Safer

2012 CRE Toolkit
http://www.cdc.gov/hai/organisms/cre/cre-toolkit/index.html

MMWR, March 2013
http://www.cdc.gov/mmwr/preview/mmwrhtml/mm6209a3.html?s_cid=mm6209a3_w

Get Smart for Healthcare
http://www.cdc.gov/getsmart/healthcare

Carbapenem-resistant Enterobacteriaceae (CRE) Resources
http://www.cdc.gov/HAI/organisms/cre/index.html

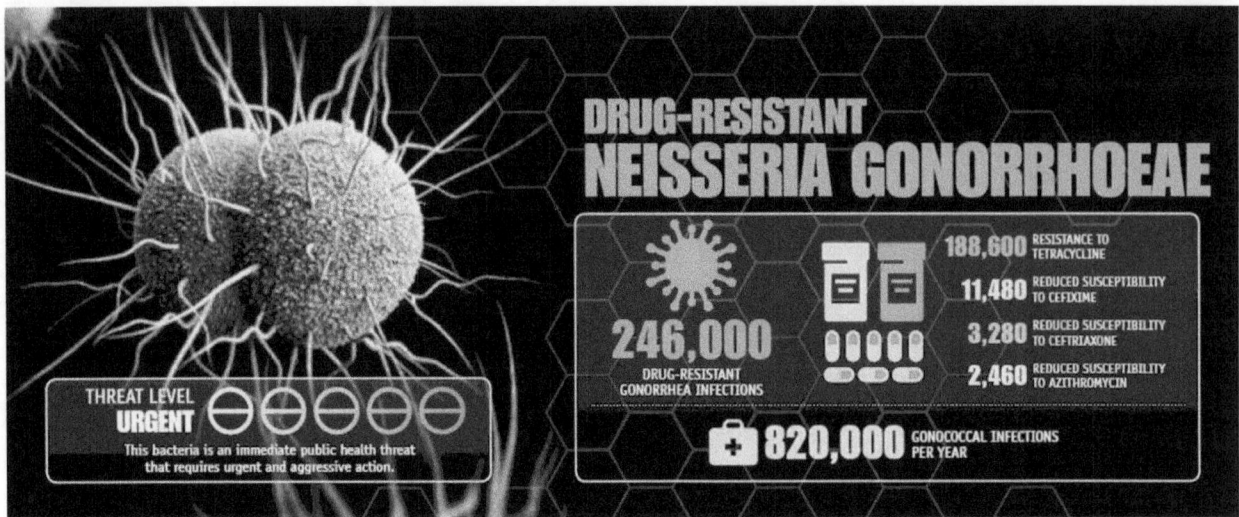

Neisseria gonorrhoeae causes gonorrhea, a sexually transmitted disease that can result in discharge and inflammation at the urethra, cervix, pharynx, or rectum.

RESISTANCE OF CONCERN

N. gonorrhoeae is showing resistance to antibiotics usually used to treat it. These drugs include:

- cefixime (an oral cephalosporin)
- ceftriaxone (an injectable cephalosporin)
- azithromycin
- tetracycline

PUBLIC HEALTH THREAT

Gonorrhea is the second most commonly reported notifiable infection in the United States and is easily transmitted. It causes severe reproductive complications and disproportionately affects sexual, racial, and ethnic minorities. Gonorrhea control relies on prompt identification and treatment of infected persons and their sex partners. Because some drugs are less effective in treating gonorrhea, CDC recently updated its treatment guidelines to slow the emergence of drug resistance. CDC now recommends only ceftriaxone plus either azithromycin or doxycycline as first-line treatment for gonorrhea. The emergence of cephalosporin resistance, especially ceftriaxone resistance, would greatly limit treatment options and could cripple gonorrhea control efforts.

In 2011, 321,849 cases of gonorrhea were reported to CDC, but CDC estimates that more than 800,000 cases occur annually in the United States.

	Percentage	Estimated number of cases
Gonorrhea		820,000
Resistance to any antibiotic	30%	246,000
Reduced susceptibility to cefixime	<1%	11,480
Reduced susceptibility to ceftriaxone	<1%	3,280
Reduced susceptibility to azithromycin	<1%	2,460
Resistance to tetracycline	23%	188,600

Source: The Gonococcal Isolate Surveillance Project (GISP)–5,900 isolates tested for susceptibility in 2011. For more information about data methods and references, please see technical appendix.

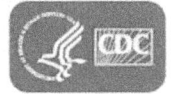

U.S. Department of Health and Human Services
Centers for Disease Control and Prevention

DRUG-RESISTANT
NEISSERIA GONORRHOEAE

FIGHTING THE SPREAD OF RESISTANCE

Cephalosporin-resistant *N. gonorrhoeae* is often resistant to multiple classes of other antibiotics and as a result, infections caused by these bacteria will likely fail empiric treatment regimens. If cephalosporin-resistant *N. gonorrhoeae* becomes widespread, the public health impact during a 10-year period is estimated to be 75,000 additional cases of pelvic inflammatory disease (a major cause of infertility), 15,000 cases of epididymitis, and 222 additional HIV infections because HIV is transmitted more readily when someone is co-infected with gonorrhea. In addition, the estimated direct medical costs would total $235 million. Additional costs are anticipated to be incurred as a result of increased susceptibility monitoring, provider education, case management, and the need for additional courses of antibiotics and follow-up.

Gonorrhea is a global problem, requiring a global approach. Action in the United States alone is unlikely to prevent resistance from developing, but rapid detection and effective treatment of patients and their partners might slow the spread of resistance. Preventing gonorrhea is critical. Screening, rapid detection, prompt treatment, and partner services are the foundations of gonorrhea control in the United States. Effectively addressing the heavy burden of gonorrhea and anticipated arrival of cephalosporin resistance requires continued use of these strategies as well as the use of expedited partner therapy, promotion of safer sexual behaviors such as abstinence, mutual monogamy, and correct and consistent condom use, and activities designed to rapidly detect and respond to antibiotic-resistant infections

WHAT CDC IS DOING

CDC is closely monitoring resistance in *N. gonorrhoeae* in the United States and actively collaborating with the World Health Organization to enhance global surveillance. In the United States, CDC recently released a national response plan and is working closely with local and state STD programs to enhance preparedness. CDC recently updated its gonorrhea treatment recommendations to stay a step ahead of this rapidly evolving bacterium, and is collaborating with the NIH National Institute of Allergy and Infectious Diseases to find new treatment options.

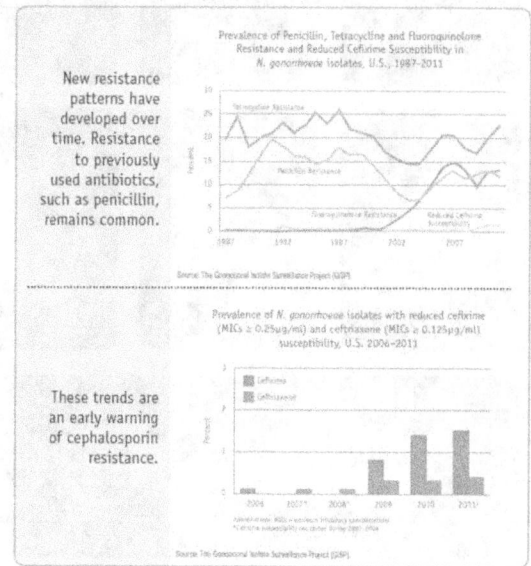

New resistance patterns have developed over time. Resistance to previously used antibiotics, such as penicillin, remains common.

These trends are an early warning of cephalosporin resistance.

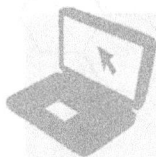

ONLINE RESOURCES

CDC's gonorrhea website
http://www.cdc.gov/std/gonorrhea/default.htm

CDC's Antibiotic-Resistant Gonorrhea website:
http://www.cdc.gov/std/Gonorrhea/arg/default.htm

New Treatment Guidelines for Gonorrhea: Antibiotic Change. MedScape CDC Expert Commentary, 2012. http://www.medscape.com/viewarticle/768883

Kirkcaldy RD, Bolan GA, Wasserheit JN. Cephalosporin-Resistant Gonorrhea in North America. JAMA 2013;209(2):185-187.
http://jama.jamanetwork.com/article.aspx?articleid=1556135

CDC. Update to CDC's Sexually Transmitted Diseases Treatment Guidelines, 2010: Oral cephalosporins no longer a recommended treatment for gonococcal infections. MMWR 2012;61(31):590-594.
http://www.cdc.gov/mmwr/preview/mmwrhtml/mm6131a3.htm?

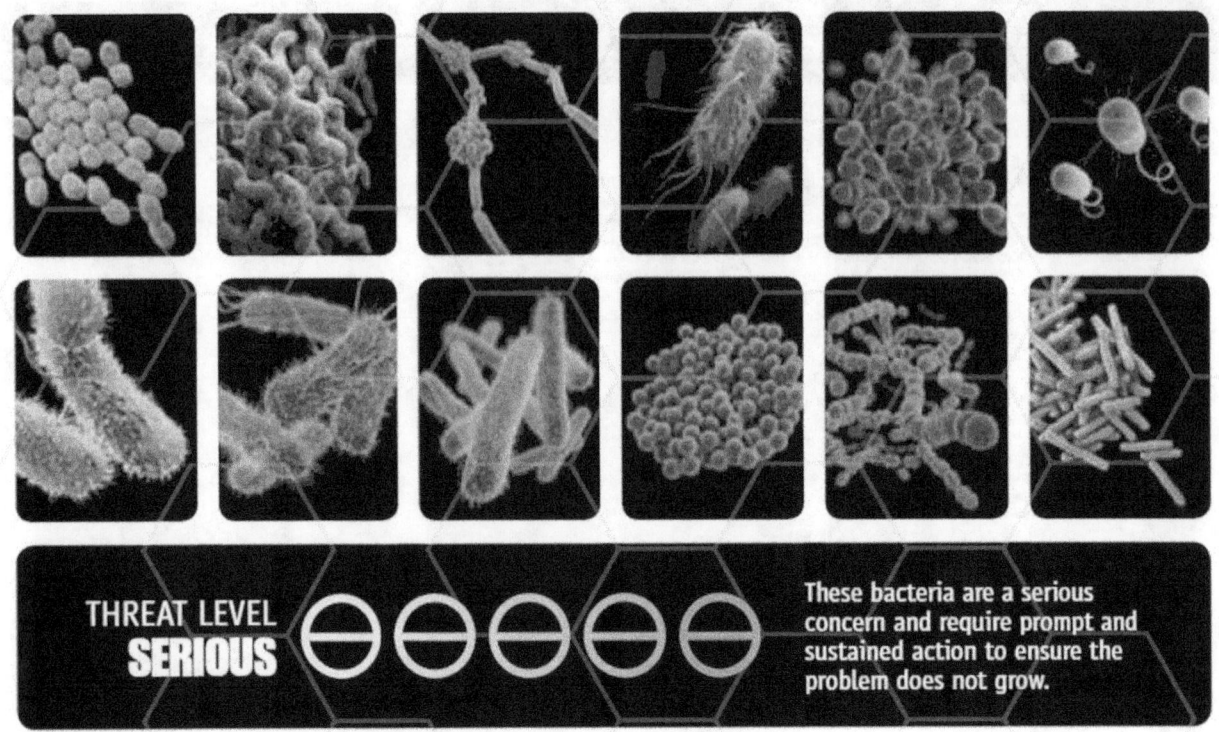

THREAT LEVEL **SERIOUS** ⊖ ⊖ ⊖ ⊖ ⊖

These bacteria are a serious concern and require prompt and sustained action to ensure the problem does not grow.

MICROORGANISMS WITH A THREAT LEVEL OF SERIOUS

Multidrug-resistant *Acinetobacter*

Drug-resistant *Campylobacter*

Fluconazole-resistant *Candida* (a fungus)

Extended spectrum β-lactamase producing **Enterobacteriaceae (ESBLs)**

Vancomycin-resistant *Enterococcus* **(VRE)**

Multidrug-resistant *Pseudomonas aeruginosa*

Drug-resistant **non-typhoidal** *Salmonella*

Drug-resistant *Salmonella* Typhi

Drug-resistant *Shigella*

Methicillin-resistant *Staphylococcus aureus* (MRSA)

Drug-resistant *Streptococcus pneumoniae*

Drug-resistant **tuberculosis**

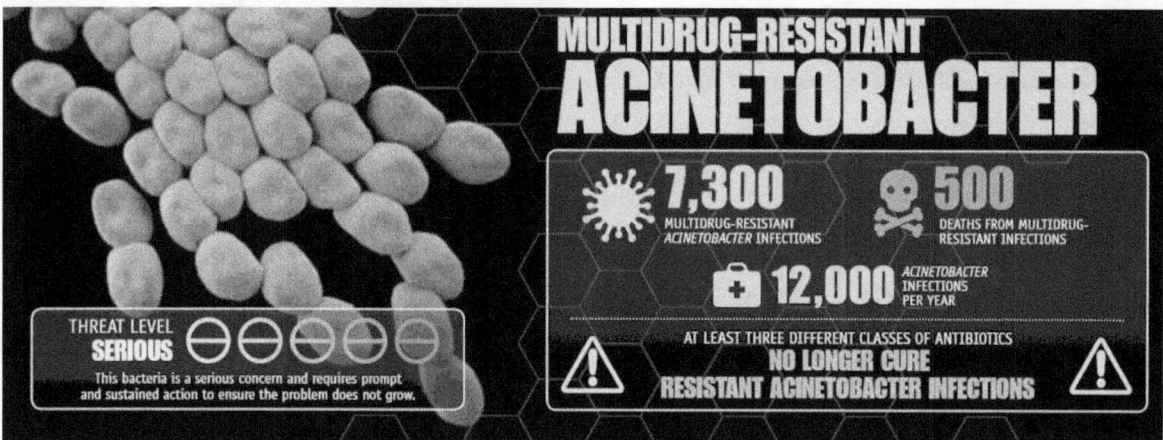

MULTIDRUG-RESISTANT
ACINETOBACTER

7,300
MULTIDRUG-RESISTANT
ACINETOBACTER INFECTIONS

500
DEATHS FROM MULTIDRUG-
RESISTANT INFECTIONS

12,000
ACINETOBACTER
INFECTIONS
PER YEAR

AT LEAST THREE DIFFERENT CLASSES OF ANTIBIOTICS
NO LONGER CURE
RESISTANT ACINETOBACTER INFECTIONS

THREAT LEVEL
SERIOUS
This bacteria is a serious concern and requires prompt
and sustained action to ensure the problem does not grow.

Acinetobacter is a type of gram-negative bacteria that is a cause of pneumonia or bloodstream infections among critically ill patients. Many of these bacteria have become very resistant to antibiotics.

RESISTANCE OF CONCERN

Some *Acinetobacter* strains are resistant to nearly all or all antibiotics including carbapenems, often considered antibiotics of last resort.

- About 63% of *Acinetobacter* is considered multidrug-resistant, meaning at least three different classes of antibiotics no longer cure *Acinetobacter* infections.

- Approximately 2% of healthcare-associated infections reported to CDC's National Healthcare Safety Network are caused by *Acinetobacter*, but the proportion is higher among critically ill patients on mechanical ventilators (about 7%).

PUBLIC HEALTH THREAT

An estimated 12,000 healthcare-associated *Acinetobacter* infections occur in the United States each year. Nearly 7,000 (or 63%) of these are multidrug-resistant, and about 500 deaths are attributed to these infections.

	Percentage of all *Acinetobacter* healthcare-associated infections that are multidrug-resistant	Estimated number of infections	Estimated number of deaths attributed
Multidrug-resistant *Acinetobacter*	63%	7,300	500

For more information about data methods and references, please see technical appendix.

MULTIDRUG-RESISTANT ACINETOBACTER

FIGHTING THE SPREAD OF RESISTANCE

WHAT CDC IS DOING

- Tracking illness and identifying risk factors for drug-resistant infections using two systems, the National Healthcare Safety Network and the Emerging Infections Program.
- Providing outbreak support such as staff expertise, prevention guidelines, tools, and lab assistance, to states and facilities.
- Developing tests and prevention recommendations to control drug-resistant infections.
- Helping medical facilities improve antibiotic prescribing practices.

WHAT YOU CAN DO

States and Communities Can:

- Know resistance trends in your region.
- Coordinate local and regional infection tracking and control efforts.
- Require facilities to alert each other when transferring patients with any infection.

Healthcare CEOs, Medical Officers, and other Healthcare Facility Leaders Can:

- Require and strictly enforce CDC guidance for infection detection, prevention, tracking, and reporting.
- Make sure your lab can accurately identify infections and alert clinical and infection prevention staff when these bacteria are present.
- Know infection and resistance trends in your facility and in the facilities around you.
- When transferring a patient, require staff to notify the other facility about all infections.
- Join or start regional infection prevention efforts.
- Promote wise antibiotic use.

Healthcare Providers Can:

- Know the type of drug-resistant infections that are present in your facility and patients.
    - Request immediate alerts when the lab identifies drug-resistant infections in your patients.
    - Alert the other facility when you transfer a patient with a drug-resistant infection.
- Protect patients from drug-resistant infections.
    - Follow relevant guidelines and precautions at every patient encounter.
    - Prescribe antibiotics wisely.
    - Remove temporary medical devices such as catheters and ventilators as soon as no longer needed.

Patients and Their Loved Ones Can:

- Ask everyone including doctors, nurses, other medical staff, and visitors, to wash their hands before touching the patient.
- Take antibiotics exactly as prescribed.

ONLINE RESOURCES

Acinetobacter in Healthcare Settings
http://www.cdc.gov/HAI/organisms/acinetobacter.html

Healthcare-associated Infections, Guidelines and Recommendations
http://www.cdc.gov/HAI/prevent/prevent_pubs.html

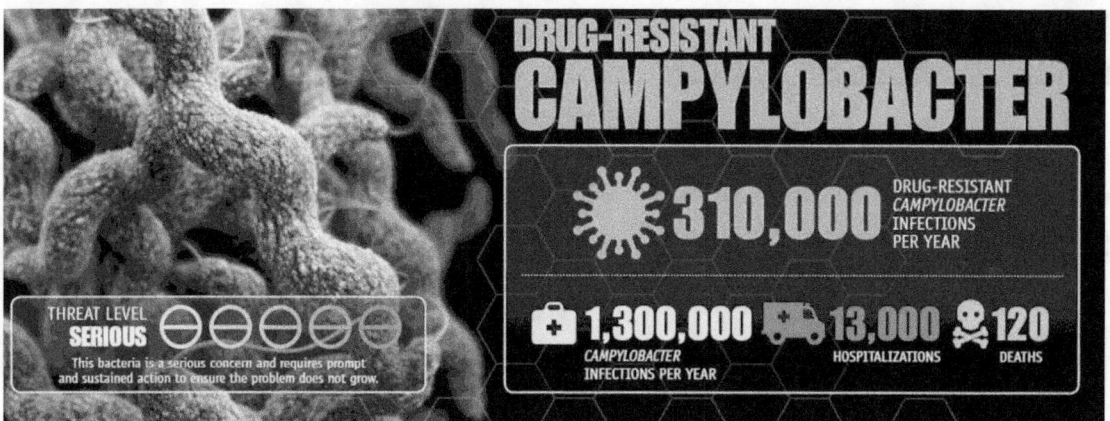

DRUG-RESISTANT CAMPYLOBACTER

310,000 DRUG-RESISTANT *CAMPYLOBACTER* INFECTIONS PER YEAR

1,300,000 *CAMPYLOBACTER* INFECTIONS PER YEAR

13,000 HOSPITALIZATIONS

120 DEATHS

THREAT LEVEL
SERIOUS
This bacteria is a serious concern and requires prompt and sustained action to ensure the problem does not grow.

Campylobacter usually causes diarrhea (often bloody), fever, and abdominal cramps, and sometimes causes serious complications such as temporary paralysis.

RESISTANCE OF CONCERN

Physicians rely on drugs like ciprofloxacin and azithromycin for treating patients with severe disease. Resistant infections sometimes last longer. *Campylobacter* is showing resistance to:

- ciprofloxacin
- azithromycin

PUBLIC HEALTH THREAT

Campylobacter is estimated to cause approximately 1.3 million infections, 13,000 hospitalizations, and 120 deaths each year in the United States. CDC is seeing resistance to ciprofloxacin in almost 25% of *Campylobacter* tested and resistance to azithromycin in about 2%. Costs are expected to be higher for resistant infections because antibiotic-resistant *Campylobacter* infections sometimes last longer.

	Percentage of all *Campylobacter**	Estimated number of illnesses per year	Estimated illnesses per 100,000 U.S. population	Estimated number of deaths per year
Resistance to ciprofloxacin	23%	310,000	102.3	28
Resistance to azithromycin	2%	22,000	7.4	<5
Resistance to azithromycin or ciprofloxacin	24%	310,000	103.9	28

Campylobacter drug resistance increased from 13% in 1997 to almost 25% in 2011.

Increasing Resistance to Ciprofloxacin in *Campylobacter*, 1989–2011

*3-year average (2009–2011)

*Data for 1989–1990 were from a sentinel county survey. Annual testing began in 1997

For more information about data methods and references, please see appendix.

FIGHTING THE SPREAD OF RESISTANCE

Campylobacter spreads from animals to people through contaminated food, particularly raw or undercooked chicken and unpasteurized milk. Infections may also be acquired through contact with animals and by drinking contaminated water. Antibiotic use in food animals can result in resistant *Campylobacter* that can spread to humans. Resistant *Campylobacter* are common in many countries and cause illness in travelers. Key measures to prevent resistant infections include:

- Avoiding inappropriate antibiotic use in food animals.
- Tracking antibiotic use in different types of food animals.
- Stopping spread of *Campylobacter* among animals on farms.
- Improving food production and processing to reduce contamination.
- Educating consumers and food workers about safe food handling practices.

WHAT CDC IS DOING

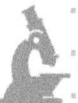

- Tracking changes in antibiotic resistance through ongoing surveillance.
- Promoting initiatives that measure and improve antibiotic use in food animals.
- Determining foods responsible for outbreaks of *Campylobacter* infections.
- Supporting and improving local, state, and federal public health surveillance.
- Guiding prevention efforts by estimating how much illness occurs and identifying the sources of infection.
- Educating people about how to avoid *Campylobacter* infections.

WHAT YOU CAN DO

- **Clean.** Wash hands, cutting boards, utensils, sinks, and countertops.
- **Separate.** Keep raw meat, poultry, and seafood separate from ready-to-eat foods.
- **Cook.** Use a food thermometer to ensure that foods are cooked to a safe internal temperature.
- **Chill.** Keep your refrigerator below 40°F and refrigerate food that will spoil.
- Avoid drinking raw milk and untreated water.
- Report suspected illness from food to your local health department.
- Don't prepare food for others if you have diarrhea or vomiting.
- Be especially careful preparing food for children, pregnant women, those in poor health, and older adults.
- Consume safe food and water when traveling abroad.

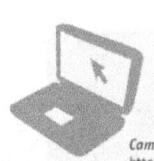

ONLINE RESOURCES

National Antimicrobial Resistance Monitoring System
http://www.cdc.gov/narms

Campylobacter **Information**
http://www.cdc.gov/nczved/divisions/dfbmd/diseases/campylobacter/

Traveler's Health
http://wwwnc.cdc.gov/travel/yellowbook/2012/chapter-2-the-pre-travel-consultation/travelers-diarrhea.htm

Vital Signs, June 2011: Making Food Safer to Eat
http://www.cdc.gov/VitalSigns/FoodSafety/

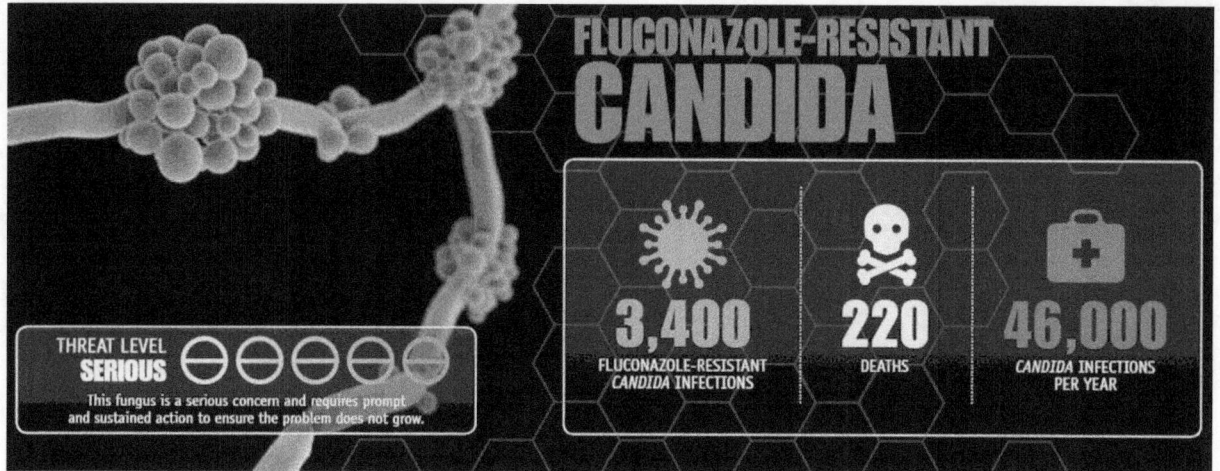

3,400
FLUCONAZOLE-RESISTANT
CANDIDA INFECTIONS

220
DEATHS

46,000
CANDIDA INFECTIONS
PER YEAR

Candidiasis is a fungal infection caused by yeasts of the genus *Candida*. There are more than 20 species of *Candida* yeasts that can cause infection in humans, the most common of which is *Candida albicans*. *Candida* yeasts normally live on the skin and mucous membranes without causing infection. However, overgrowth of these microorganisms can cause symptoms to develop. Symptoms of candidiasis vary depending on the area of the body that is infected.

Candida is the fourth most common cause of healthcare-associated bloodstream infections in the United States. In some hospitals it is the most common cause. These infections tend to occur in the sickest of patients.

RESISTANCE OF CONCERN

- Some *Candida* strains are increasingly resistant to first-line and second-line antifungal treatment agents. Recent data demonstrate a marked shift among infections towards *Candida* species with increased resistance to antifungal drugs including azoles and echinocandins.

- CDC conducts multicenter surveillance for antifungal resistance in the United States, candidal infections, their economic impact, and possible areas where prevention and control strategies can be focused.

PUBLIC HEALTH THREAT

An estimated 46,000 healthcare-associated *Candida* infections occur among hospitalized patients in the United States each year. Roughly 30% of patients with bloodstream infections (candidemia) with drug-resistant *Candida* die during their hospitalization. CDC estimates that each case of *Candida* infection results in 3-13 days of additional hospitalization, and a total of $6,000–$29,000 in direct healthcare costs. Based on these estimates, we calculate resistant *Candida* infections may add millions of dollars in excess costs to U.S. healthcare expenditures each year.

	Percentage of Candida bloodstream isolates testing resistant	Estimated number of infections per year	Estimated number of deaths
Fluconazole-resistant *Candida* species	7%	3,400	220

For more information about data methods and references, please see technical appendix.

FIGHTING THE SPREAD OF RESISTANCE

Prevention strategies for candidemia are not well defined. Most infectious are thought to be caused by *Candida* that the patient carries on his or her own body. Therapy to prevent infections (antifungal prophylaxis) may be appropriate for some groups at high risk of developing *Candida* bloodstream infection, such as low-birth-weight infants. CDC recommendations for catheter care and handwashing can be helpful in reducing transmission in healthcare institutions.

WHAT CDC IS DOING

Prevention of significant morbidity and mortality from candidemia remains a challenge. Although antifungal prophylaxis has been shown to be effective in selected patient populations, there is still debate on the application of risk prevention tools and other prevention strategies. There is a continued need for surveillance of candidemia to develop and evaluate prevention strategies and to monitor for changes in incidence and resistance.

There is increasing incidence of *Candida* infections due to azole- and echinocandin-resistant strains.

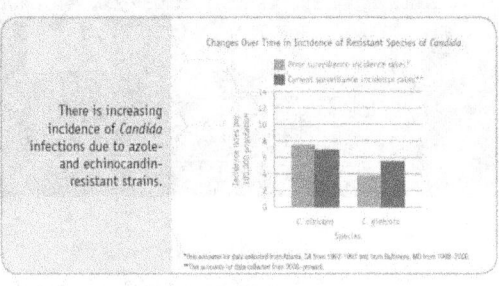

ONLINE RESOURCES

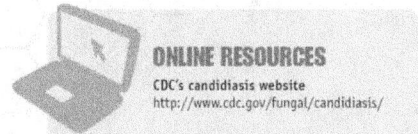

CDC's candidiasis website
http://www.cdc.gov/fungal/candidiasis/

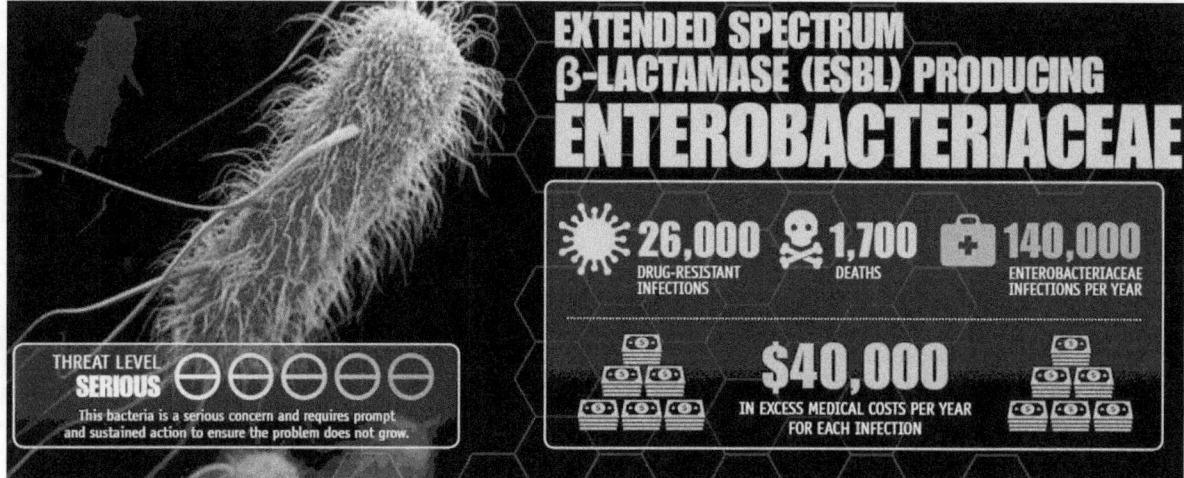

EXTENDED SPECTRUM
β-LACTAMASE (ESBL) PRODUCING
ENTEROBACTERIACEAE

26,000 DRUG-RESISTANT INFECTIONS

1,700 DEATHS

140,000 ENTEROBACTERIACEAE INFECTIONS PER YEAR

$40,000 IN EXCESS MEDICAL COSTS PER YEAR FOR EACH INFECTION

THREAT LEVEL
SERIOUS
This bacteria is a serious concern and requires prompt and sustained action to ensure the problem does not grow.

Extended-spectrum β-lactamase is an enzyme that allows bacteria to become resistant to a wide variety of penicillins and cephalosporins. Bacteria that contain this enzyme are known as ESBLs or ESBL-producing bacteria. ESBL-producing Enterobacteriaceae are resistant to strong antibiotics including extended spectrum cephalosporins.

RESISTANCE OF CONCERN

Some Enterobacteriaceae are resistant to nearly all:

- penicillins
- cephalosporins

In these cases, the remaining treatment option is an antibiotic from the carbapenem family. These are drugs of last resort, and use of them is also contributing to resistance (see CRE fact sheet).

- Nearly 26,000 (or 19%) healthcare-associated Enterobacteriaceae infections are caused by ESBL-producing Enterobacteriaceae.
- Patients with bloodstream infections caused by ESBL-producing Enterobacteriaceae are about 57% more likely to die than those with bloodstream infections caused by a non ESBL-producing strain.

PUBLIC HEALTH THREAT

An estimated 140,000 healthcare-associated Enterobacteriaceae infections occur in the United States each year. CDC estimates that bloodstream infections caused by ESBL-containing Enterobacteriaceae result in upwards of $40,000 in excess hospital charges per occurrence. Approximately 26,000 infections and 1,700 deaths are attributable to ESBLs.

	Percentage of Enterobacteriaceae healthcare-associated infections resistant to extended spectrum cephalosporins	Estimated number of infections	Estimated number of deaths attributed
ESBL-producing *Klebsiella* spp.	23%	17,000	1,100
ESBL-producing *E. coli*	14%	9,000	600
Totals		26,000	1,700

For more information about data methods and references, please see technical appendix.

153

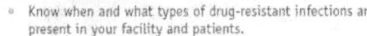
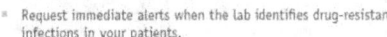

EXTENDED SPECTRUM β-LACTAMASE (ESBL) PRODUCING
ENTEROBACTERIACEAE

FIGHTING THE SPREAD OF RESISTANCE

WHAT CDC IS DOING

- Tracking illness and identifying risk factors for drug-resistant infections using two systems, the National Healthcare Safety Network and the Emerging Infections Program.
- Providing outbreak support, such as staff expertise, prevention guidelines, tools, and lab assistance, to states and facilities.
- Developing tests and prevention recommendations to control drug-resistant infections.
- Helping medical facilities improve antibiotic prescribing practices.

WHAT YOU CAN DO

States and Communities Can:

- Know resistance trends in your region.
- Coordinate local and regional infection tracking and control efforts.
- Require facilities to alert each other when transferring patients with any infection.

Health Care CEOs, Medical Officers, and Other Healthcare Facility Leaders Can:

- Require and strictly enforce CDC guidance for infection detection, prevention, tracking, and reporting.
- Make sure your lab can accurately identify infections and alert clinical and infection prevention staff when these bacteria are present.
- Know infection and resistance trends in your facility and in the facilities around you.
- When transferring a patient, require staff to notify the other facility about all infections.
- Join or start regional infection prevention efforts.
- Promote wise antibiotic use.

Healthcare Providers Can:

- Know when and what types of drug-resistant infections are present in your facility and patients.
- Request immediate alerts when the lab identifies drug-resistant infections in your patients.
- Alert the other facility when you transfer a patient with a drug-resistant infection.
- Protect patients from drug-resistant infections.
- Follow relevant guidelines and precautions at every patient encounter.
- Prescribe antibiotics wisely.
- Remove temporary medical devices such as catheters and ventilators as soon as no longer needed.

Patients and Their Loved Ones Can:

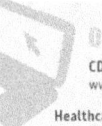

- Ask everyone including doctors, nurses, other medical staff, and visitors, to wash their hands before touching the patient.
- Take antibiotics only and exactly as prescribed.

ONLINE RESOURCES

CDC's Heathcare-associated Infections(HAI) website
www.cdc.gov/hai

Healthcare-associated Infections (HAIs), Guidelines and Recommendations
www.cdc.gov/hicpac/pubs.html

154

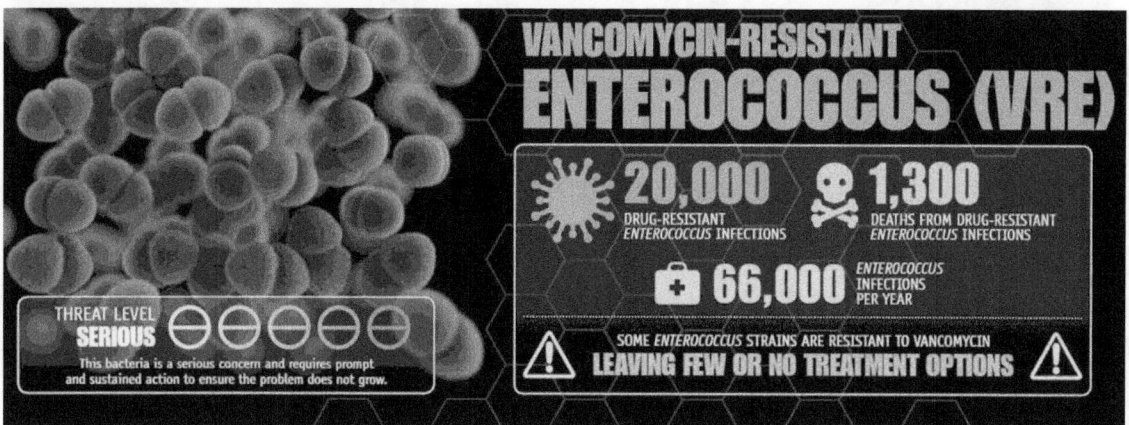

VANCOMYCIN-RESISTANT
ENTEROCOCCUS (VRE)

20,000
DRUG-RESISTANT
ENTEROCOCCUS INFECTIONS

1,300
DEATHS FROM DRUG-RESISTANT
ENTEROCOCCUS INFECTIONS

66,000
ENTEROCOCCUS
INFECTIONS
PER YEAR

THREAT LEVEL
SERIOUS
This bacteria is a serious concern and requires prompt
and sustained action to ensure the problem does not grow.

SOME *ENTEROCOCCUS* STRAINS ARE RESISTANT TO VANCOMYCIN
⚠ **LEAVING FEW OR NO TREATMENT OPTIONS** ⚠

Enterococci cause a range of illnesses, mostly among patients receiving healthcare, but include bloodstream infections, surgical site infections, and urinary tract infections.

RESISTANCE OF CONCERN

- *Enterococcus* often cause infections among very sick patients in hospitals and other healthcare-settings.
- Some *Enterococcus* strains are resistant to vancomycin, an antibiotic of last resort, leaving few or no treatment options.
- About 20,000 (or 30%) of *Enterococcus* healthcare-associated infections are vancomycin resistant.

PUBLIC HEALTH THREAT

An estimated 66,000 healthcare-associated *Enterococcus* infections occur in the United States each year. The proportion of infections that occur with a vancomycin resistant strain differs by the species of *Enterococcus;* overall 20,000 vancomycin-resistant infections occurred among hospitalized patients each year, with approximately 1,300 deaths attributed to these infections.

	Percent of all *Enterococcus* healthcare-associated infections resistant to vancomycin	Estimated number of infections	Estimated number of deaths attributed
Vancomycin-resistant *Enterococcus faecium*	77%	10,000	650
Vancomycin-resistant *Enterococcus faecalis*	9%	3,100	200
Vancomycin-resistant *Enterococcus* (species not determined)	40%	6,900	450
Totals		20,000	1,300

For more information about data methods and references, please see technical appendix

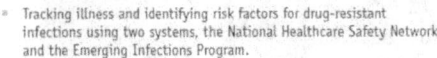

VANCOMYCIN-RESISTANT ENTEROCOCCUS (VRE)

FIGHTING THE SPREAD OF RESISTANCE

WHAT CDC IS DOING

- Tracking illness and identifying risk factors for drug-resistant infections using two systems, the National Healthcare Safety Network and the Emerging Infections Program.
- Providing outbreak support such as staff expertise, prevention guidelines, tools, and lab assistance, to states and facilities.
- Developing tests and prevention recommendations to control drug-resistant infections.
- Helping medical facilities improve antibiotic prescribing practices.

WHAT YOU CAN DO

States and Communities can:

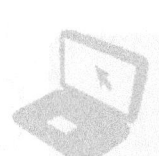

- Know resistance trends in your region.
- Coordinate local and regional infection tracking and control efforts.
- Require facilities to alert each other when transferring patients with any infection.

Healthcare CEOs, Medical Officers, and other Healthcare Facility Leaders can:

- Require and strictly enforce CDC guidance for infection detection, prevention, tracking, and reporting.
- Make sure your lab can accurately identify infections and alert clinical and infection prevention staff when these germs are present.
- Know infection and resistance trends in your facility and in the facilities around you.
- When transferring a patient, require staff to notify the other facility about all infections.
- Join or start regional infection prevention efforts.
- Promote wise antibiotic use.

Doctors and Nurses can:

- Know when and what types of drug-resistant infections are present in your facility and patients Request immediate alerts when the lab identifies drug-resistant infections in your patients.
- Alert the other facility when you transfer a patient with a drug-resistant infection.
- Protect patients from drug-resistant infections.
- Follow relevant guidelines and precautions at every patient encounter.
- Prescribe antibiotics wisely.
- Remove temporary medical devices such as catheters and ventilators as soon as no longer needed.

Patients and their loved ones can:

- Ask everyone including doctors, nurses, other medical staff, and visitors, to wash their hands before touching the patient.
- Take antibiotics only and exactly as prescribed.

ONLINE RESOURCES

Vancomycin-resistant Enterococci (VRE) in Healthcare Settings
http://www.cdc.gov/HAI/organisms/vre/vre.html

Healthcare-associated Infections (HAIs), Guidelines and Recommendations
www.cdc.gov/hicpac/pubs.html

156

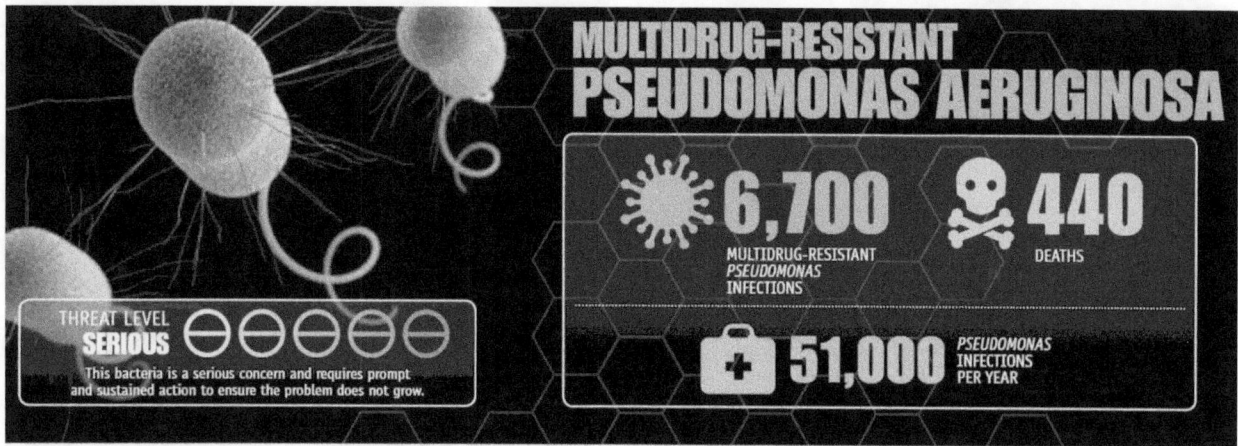

Pseudomonas aeruginosa is a common cause of healthcare-associated infections including pneumonia, bloodstream infections, urinary tract infections, and surgical site infections.

RESISTANCE OF CONCERN

- Some strains of *Pseudomonas aeruginosa* have been found to be resistant to nearly all or all antibiotics including aminoglycosides, cephalosporins, fluoroquinolones, and carbapenems.

- Approximately 8% of all healthcare-associated infections reported to CDC's National Healthcare Safety Network are caused by *Pseudomonas aeruginosa*.

- About 13% of severe healthcare-associated infections caused by *Pseudomonas aeruginosa* are multidrug resistant, meaning several classes of antibiotics no longer cure these infections.

PUBLIC HEALTH THREAT

An estimated 51,000 healthcare-associated *Pseudomonas aeruginosa* infections occur in the United States each year. More than 6,000 (or 13%) of these are multidrug-resistant, with roughly 400 deaths per year attributed to these infections.

	Percentage of all *Pseudomonas aeruginosa* healthcare-associated infections that are multidrug-resistant	Estimated number of infections	Estimated number of deaths attributed
Multi-drug resistant *Pseudomonas aeruginosa*	13%	6,700	440

For more information about data methods and references, please see technical appendix.

MULTIDRUG-RESISTANT
PSEUDOMONAS AERUGINOSA

FIGHTING THE SPREAD OF RESISTANCE

WHAT CDC IS DOING

- Identifying and tracking risk factors for drug-resistant infections using two systems, the National Healthcare Safety Network and the Emerging Infections Program.
- Providing outbreak support such as staff expertise, prevention guidelines, tools, and lab assistance, to states and facilities.
- Developing tests and prevention recommendations to control drug-resistant infections.
- Helping medical facilities improve antibiotic prescribing practices.

WHAT YOU CAN DO

States and Communities Can:

- Know resistance trends in your region.
- Coordinate local and regional infection tracking and control efforts.
- Require facilities to alert each other when transferring patients with any infection.

Health Care CEOs, Medical Officers, and Other Healthcare Facility Leaders Can:

- Require and strictly enforce CDC guidance for infection detection, prevention, tracking, and reporting.
- Make sure your lab can accurately identify infections and alert clinical and infection prevention staff when these bacteria are present.
- Know infection and resistance trends in your facility and in the facilities around you.
- When transferring a patient, require staff to notify the other facility about all infections.
- Join or start regional infection prevention efforts.
- Promote wise antibiotic use.

Healthcare Providers Can:

- Know when and what types of drug-resistant infections that are present in your facility and patients.
- Request immediate alerts when the lab identifies drug-resistant infections in your patients.
- Alert the other facility when you transfer a patient with a drug-resistant infection.
- Protect patients from drug-resistant infections.
- Follow relevant guidelines and precautions at every patient encounter.
- Prescribe antibiotics wisely.
- Remove temporary medical devices such as catheters and ventilators as soon as no longer needed.

Patients and Their Loved Ones Can:

- Ask everyone including doctors, nurses, other medical staff, and visitors, to wash their hands before touching the patient.
- Take antibiotics only and exactly as prescribed.

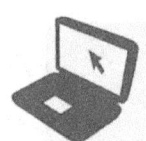

ONLINE RESOURCES

Healthcare-associated Infections (HAI)
www.cdc.gov/hai

Healthcare-associated Infections (HAIs), Guidelines and Recommendations
www.cdc.gov/hicpac/pubs.html

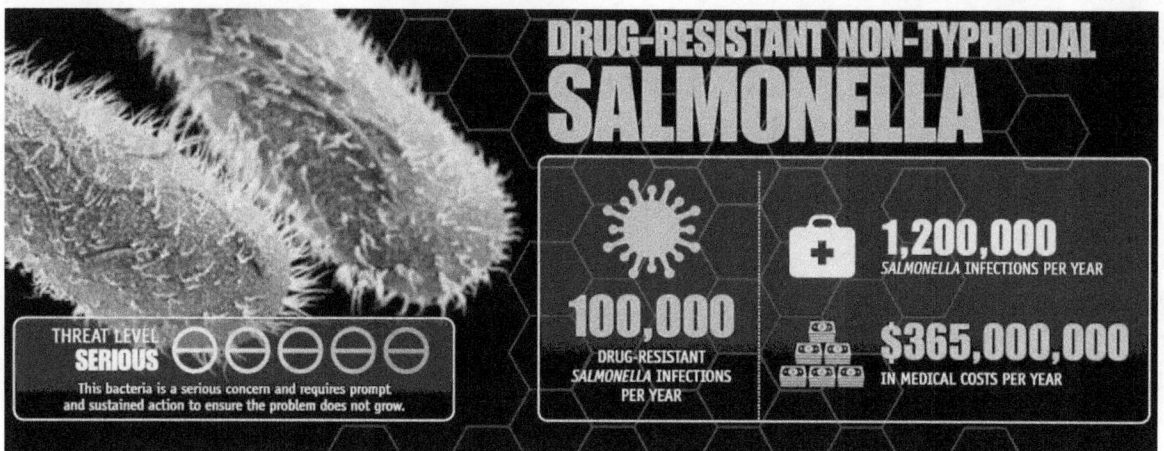

DRUG-RESISTANT NON-TYPHOIDAL SALMONELLA

THREAT LEVEL SERIOUS ⊖⊖⊖⊖⊖
This bacteria is a serious concern and requires prompt and sustained action to ensure the problem does not grow.

100,000 DRUG-RESISTANT *SALMONELLA* INFECTIONS PER YEAR

1,200,000 *SALMONELLA* INFECTIONS PER YEAR

$365,000,000 IN MEDICAL COSTS PER YEAR

Non-typhoidal *Salmonella* (serotypes other than Typhi, Paratyphi A, Paratyphi B, and Paratyphi C) usually causes diarrhea (sometimes bloody), fever, and abdominal cramps. Some infections spread to the blood and can have life-threatening complications.

RESISTANCE OF CONCERN

Physicians rely on drugs, such as ceftriaxone and ciprofloxacin, for treating patients with complicated *Salmonella* infections. Resistant infections are more severe and have higher hospitalization rates. Non-typhoidal *Salmonella* is showing resistance to:

- ceftriaxone
- ciprofloxacin
- multiple classes of drugs

PUBLIC HEALTH THREAT

Non-typhoidal *Salmonella* causes approximately 1.2 million illnesses, 23,000 hospitalizations, and 450 deaths each year in the United States. Direct medical costs are estimated to be $365 million annually. CDC is seeing resistance to ceftriaxone in about 3% of non-typhoidal *Salmonella* tested, and some level of resistance to ciprofloxacin in about 3%. About 5% of non-typhoidal *Salmonella* tested by CDC are resistant to five or more types of drugs. Costs are expected to be higher for resistant than for susceptible infections because resistant infections are more severe, those patients are more likely to be hospitalized, and treatment is less effective.

	Percentage of all non-typhoidal *Salmonella**	Estimated number of illnesses per year	Estimated illnesses per 100,000 U.S. population	Estimated number of deaths per year
Ceftriaxone resistance	3%	36,000	12.0	13
Ciprofloxacin resistance or partial resistance	3%	33,000	10.9	12
Resistance to 5 or more antibiotic classes	5%	66,000	21.9	24
Any resistance pattern above	8%	100,000	34.1	38

*3-year average (2009–2011)
For more information about data methods and references, please see technical appendix.

159

FIGHTING THE SPREAD OF RESISTANCE

Salmonella spreads from animals to people mostly through food. Antibiotic use in food animals can result in resistant *Salmonella*, and people get sick when they eat foods contaminated with *Salmonella*. Key measures to prevent resistant infections include:

- Avoiding inappropriate antibiotic use in food animals.
- Tracking antibiotic use in different types of food animals.
- Stopping spread of *Salmonella* among animals on farms.
- Improving food production and processing to reduce contamination.
- Educating consumers and food workers about safe food handling practices.

WHAT CDC IS DOING

- Tracking changes in antibiotic resistance through ongoing surveillance.
- Promoting initiatives that measure and improve antibiotic use in food animals.
- Determining foods responsible for outbreaks of *Salmonella* infections.
- Supporting and improving local, state, and federal public health surveillance.
- Guiding prevention efforts by estimating how much illness occurs and identifying the sources of infection.
- Educating people about how to avoid *Salmonella* infections.

WHAT YOU CAN DO

- **Clean.** Wash hands, cutting boards, utensils, and countertops.
- **Separate.** Keep raw meat, poultry, and seafood separate from ready-to-eat foods.
- **Cook.** Use a food thermometer to ensure that foods are cooked to a safe internal temperature.
- **Chill.** Keep your refrigerator below 40°F and refrigerate food that will spoil.

- Avoid drinking raw milk.
- Report suspected illness from food to your local health department.
- Don't prepare food for others if you have diarrhea or vomiting.
- Be especially careful preparing food for children, pregnant women, those in poor health, and older adults.

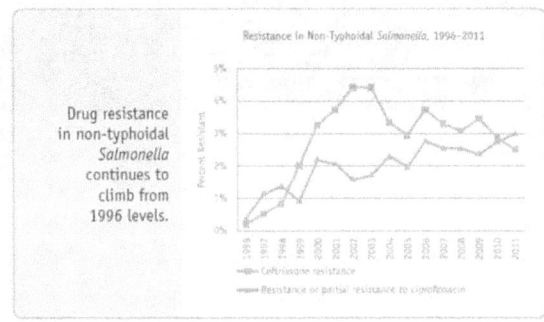

Drug resistance in non-typhoidal *Salmonella* continues to climb from 1996 levels.

For more information about data methods and references, please see appendix.

ONLINE RESOURCES

National Antimicrobial Resistance Monitoring System
http://www.cdc.gov/narms

Salmonella
http://www.cdc.gov/salmonella/index.html

Vital Signs, June 2011: Making Food Safer to Eat
http://www.cdc.gov/VitalSigns/FoodSafety/?pkw=vs_fs009

160

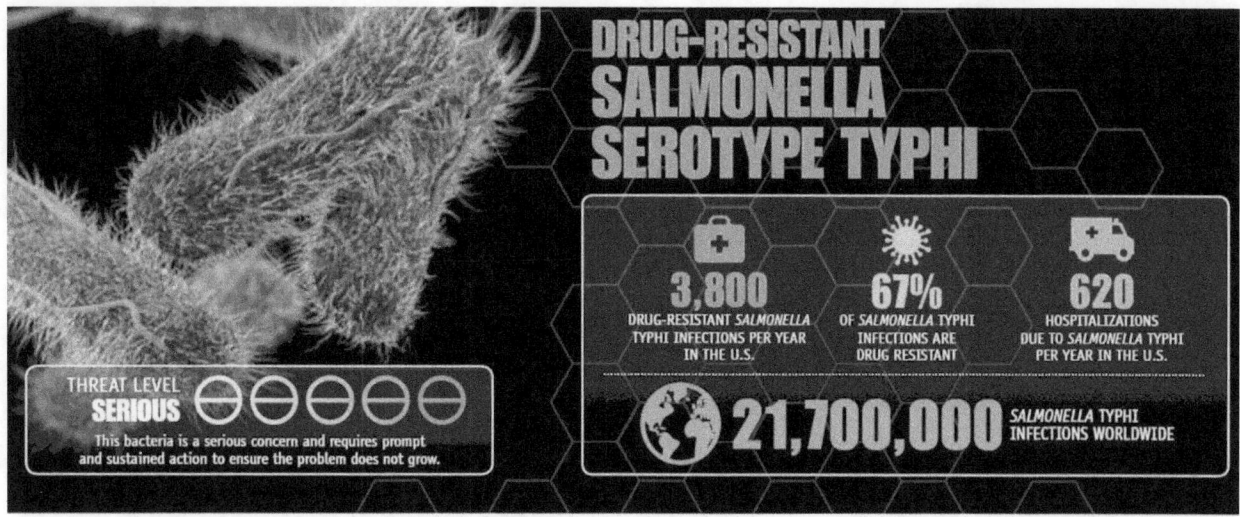

DRUG-RESISTANT
SALMONELLA
SEROTYPE TYPHI

3,800
DRUG-RESISTANT *SALMONELLA*
TYPHI INFECTIONS PER YEAR
IN THE U.S.

67%
OF *SALMONELLA* TYPHI
INFECTIONS ARE
DRUG RESISTANT

620
HOSPITALIZATIONS
DUE TO *SALMONELLA* TYPHI
PER YEAR IN THE U.S.

21,700,000 *SALMONELLA* TYPHI
INFECTIONS WORLDWIDE

THREAT LEVEL
SERIOUS ⊖⊖⊖⊖⊖
This bacteria is a serious concern and requires prompt
and sustained action to ensure the problem does not grow.

Salmonella serotype Typhi causes typhoid fever, a potentially life-threatening disease. People with typhoid fever usually have a high fever, abdominal pain, and headache. Typhoid fever can lead to bowel perforation, shock, and death.

RESISTANCE OF CONCERN

Physicians rely on drugs such as ceftriaxone, azithromycin, and ciprofloxacin for treating patients with typhoid fever. *Salmonella* serotype Typhi is showing resistance to:

- ceftriaxone
- azithromycin
- ciprofloxacin (resistance is so common that it cannot be routinely used)

PUBLIC HEALTH THREAT

Salmonella Typhi causes approximately 21.7 million illnesses worldwide. In the United States, it causes approximately 5,700 illnesses and 620 hospitalizations each year. Most illnesses occur in people who travel to some parts of the developing world where the disease is common. Travel-associated infections are more likely to be antibiotic resistant. CDC is seeing some level of resistance to ciprofloxacin in two-thirds of *Salmonella* Typhi tested. CDC has not yet seen resistance to ceftriaxone or azithromycin in the United States, but this has been seen in other parts of the world. Resistant infections are likely to cost

more than susceptible infections because illness may last longer. Deaths in the United States are rare now, but before there were antibiotics, 10% to 20% of patients died.

	Percentage of all *Salmonella* Typhi*	Estimated number of illnesses per year	Estimated illnesses per 100,000 U.S. population	Estimated number of deaths per year
Resistance or partial resistance to ciprofloxacin	67%	3,800	1.3	<5

*3-year average (2009–2011)
For more information about data methods and references, please see technical appendix.

DRUG-RESISTANT
SALMONELLA SEROTYPE TYPHI

FIGHTING THE SPREAD OF RESISTANCE

Salmonella serotype Typhi spreads from one person to another through food or water contaminated with feces. Typhoid fever is common in developing countries lacking safe water and adequate sanitation. Most U.S. cases are associated with travel to those countries. Sometimes the source is a carrier who is no longer ill, but is still infected. Key measures to prevent the spread of resistant infections include:

- Vaccinating people traveling to countries where typhoid fever is common.
- Consuming safe food and water when traveling in those countries.
- Improving access to clean water and sanitation for people living in those countries.
- Reporting changes in resistance to people who diagnose and treat patients with typhoid fever.
- Investigating cases of typhoid fever to identify and treat carriers.

WHAT CDC IS DOING

- Providing recommendations for travelers on vaccination, safe food, and clean water.
- Tracking and reporting changes in antibiotic resistance through ongoing surveillance.
- Determining settings and high-risk groups for resistant infections in the U.S. and other countries.
- Educating healthcare providers about specific resistance problems and the need to vaccinate travelers.
- Promoting safer water and sanitation in countries where typhoid fever is common.
- Building public health capacity in other countries to diagnose, track, and control typhoid fever.

ONLINE RESOURCES

National Antimicrobial Resistance Monitoring System
http://www.cdc.gov/narms

Typhoid Fever
http://www.cdc.gov/nczved/divisions/dfbmd/diseases/typhoid_fever/

Traveler's Health "Traveler's Diarrhea"
http://wwwnc.cdc.gov/travel/yellowbook/2012/chapter-2-the-pre-travel-consultation/travelers-diarrhea.htm

WHAT YOU CAN DO

If you're traveling to a country where typhoid fever is common:

- Get vaccinated against typhoid fever before you depart.
- Choose foods and drinks carefully while traveling even if you are vaccinated. That means: boil it, cook it, peel it, or forget it.
  - Boil or treat water yourself.
  - Eat foods that are hot and steaming.
  - Avoid raw fruits and vegetables unless you peel them yourself.
  - Avoid cold food and beverages from street vendors.
- If you get sick with high fever and a headache during or after travel, seek medical care at once and tell the healthcare provider where you have traveled.

Drug resistance in *Salmonella* Typhi has jumped significantly—from about 20% in 1999 to more than 70% in 2011.

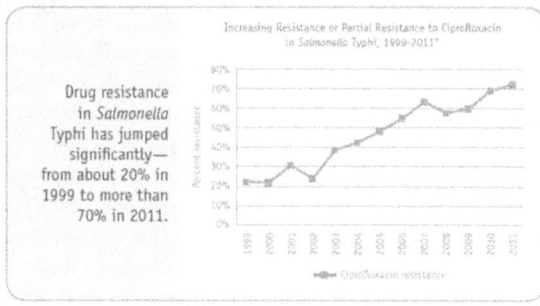

Increasing Resistance or Partial Resistance to Ciprofloxacin in *Salmonella* Typhi, 1999-2011

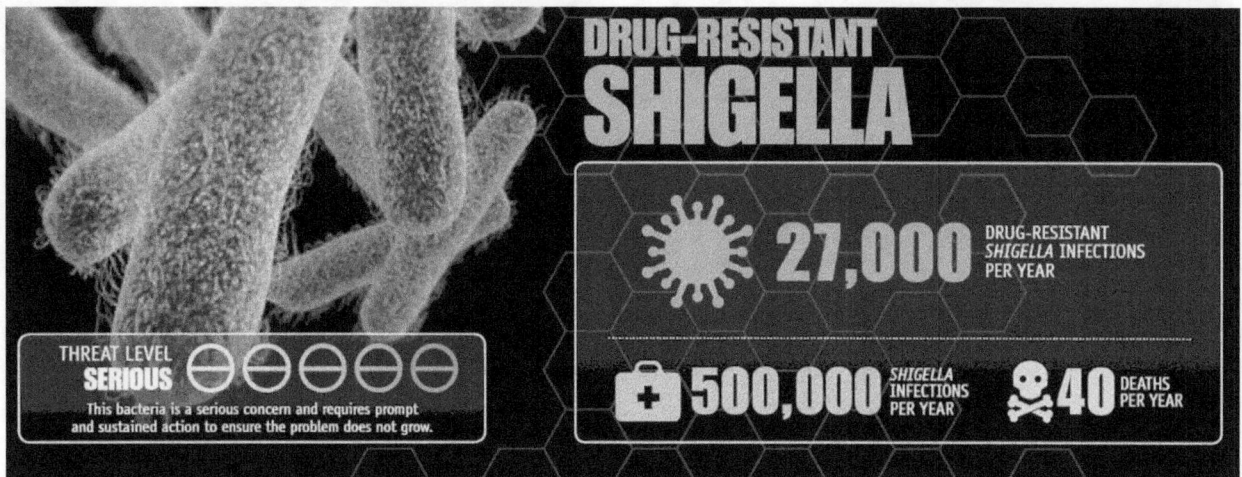

DRUG-RESISTANT SHIGELLA

27,000 DRUG-RESISTANT *SHIGELLA* INFECTIONS PER YEAR

THREAT LEVEL
SERIOUS
This bacteria is a serious concern and requires prompt and sustained action to ensure the problem does not grow.

500,000 *SHIGELLA* INFECTIONS PER YEAR

40 DEATHS PER YEAR

Shigella usually causes diarrhea (sometimes bloody), fever, and abdominal pain. Sometimes it causes serious complications such as reactive arthritis. High-risk groups include young children, people with inadequate handwashing and hygiene habits, and men who have sex with men.

RESISTANCE OF CONCERN

Resistance to traditional first-line drugs such as ampicillin and trimethoprim-sulfamethoxazole has become so high that physicians must now rely on alternative drugs like ciprofloxacin and azithromycin to treat infections. Resistant infections can last longer than infections with susceptible bacteria (bacteria that can be treated effectively with antibiotics). *Shigella* is showing resistance to:

- ciprofloxacin
- azithromycin

PUBLIC HEALTH THREAT

Shigella causes approximately 500,000 diarrheal illnesses, 5,500 hospitalizations, and 40 deaths each year in the United States. CDC is seeing resistance to ciprofloxacin in 1.6% of the *Shigella* cases tested and resistance to azithromycin in approximately 3%. Because initial treatment can fail, costs are expected to be higher for resistant infections.

	Percentage of all *Shigella**	Estimated number of illnesses per year	Estimated illnesses per 100,000 U.S. population	Estimated number of deaths per year
Ciprofloxacin resistance	2%	12,000	4.0	<5
Azithromycin resistance	3%	15,000	5.1	<5
Azithromycin or ciprofloxacin resistance	6%	27,000	9.1	<5

*Percentage of all isolates that were resistant in 2011.
For more information about data methods and references, please see technical appendix.

163

DRUG-RESISTANT
SHIGELLA

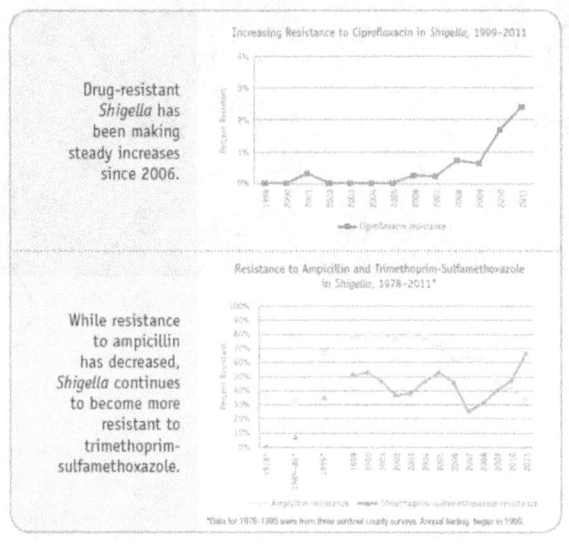

FIGHTING THE SPREAD OF RESISTANCE

Shigella spreads from one person to another in feces through direct contact, or through contaminated surfaces, food, or water. Antibiotic use in humans can result in resistant *Shigella* and hasten further spread. Key measures to prevent resistant infections include:

- Promoting thorough and frequent hand washing with soap, especially in child care centers, elementary schools, restaurants, and homes with small children.
- Using antibiotics to treat more severe *Shigella* infections and managing milder infections with fluids and rest.
- Reporting changes in resistance to healthcare providers.
- Detecting and controlling outbreaks of *Shigella* infections.
- Educating consumers and food workers about safe food handling practices.

WHAT CDC IS DOING

- Tracking changes in antibiotic resistance through ongoing surveillance.
- Determining settings and high-risk groups for outbreaks of resistant infections.
- Educating healthcare providers about specific resistance problems.
- Promoting prudent antibiotic use and handwashing.

WHAT YOU CAN DO

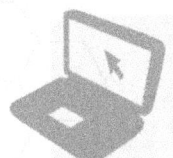

- Don't prepare food for others if you have diarrhea or vomiting.
- Keep children who have diarrhea and who are in diapers out of child care settings and swimming pools.
- Avoid sexual behavior that is likely to transmit infection when you have diarrhea.
- Consume safe food and water when traveling abroad.

Drug-resistant *Shigella* has been making steady increases since 2006.

Increasing Resistance to Ciprofloxacin in *Shigella*, 1999-2011

While resistance to ampicillin has decreased, *Shigella* continues to become more resistant to trimethoprim-sulfamethoxazole.

Resistance to Ampicillin and Trimethoprim-Sulfamethoxazole in *Shigella*, 1978-2011*

*Data for 1978-1995 were from three sentinel county surveys. Annual testing began in 1999.

ONLINE RESOURCES

National Antimicrobial Resistance Monitoring System
http://www.cdc.gov/narms

Shigellosis
http://www.cdc.gov/nczved/divisions/dfbmd/diseases/shigellosis/

Traveler's Health "Traveler's Diarrhea"
http://wwwnc.cdc.gov/travel/yellowbook/2012/chapter-2-the-pre-travel-consultation/travelers-diarrhea.htm

164

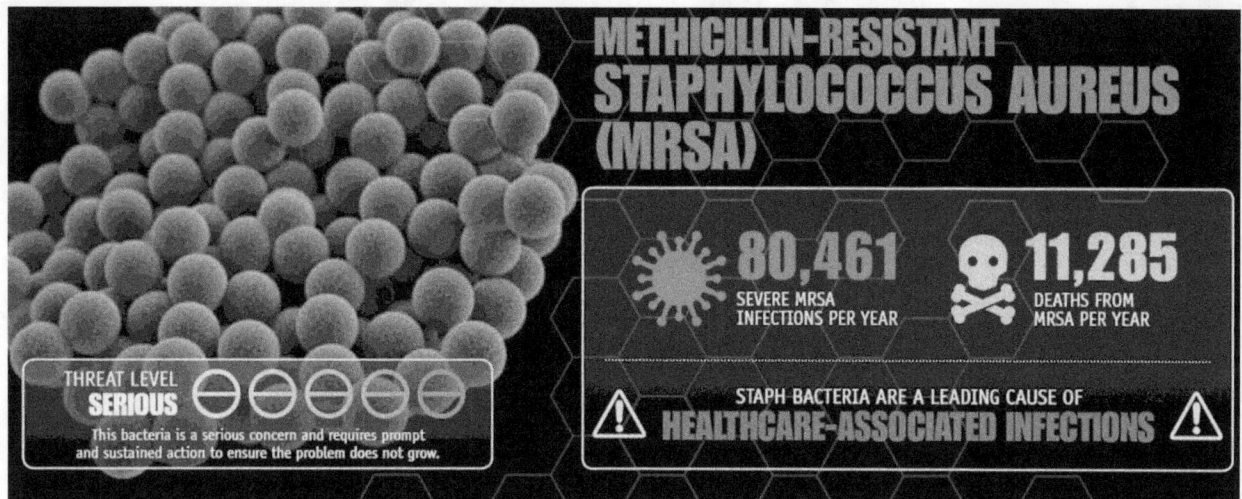

METHICILLIN-RESISTANT STAPHYLOCOCCUS AUREUS (MRSA)

80,461 SEVERE MRSA INFECTIONS PER YEAR

11,285 DEATHS FROM MRSA PER YEAR

THREAT LEVEL SERIOUS
This bacteria is a serious concern and requires prompt and sustained action to ensure the problem does not grow.

STAPH BACTERIA ARE A LEADING CAUSE OF **HEALTHCARE-ASSOCIATED INFECTIONS**

Methicillin-resistant *Staphylococcus aureus* (MRSA) causes a range of illnesses, from skin and wound infections to pneumonia and bloodstream infections that can cause sepsis and death. Staph bacteria, including MRSA, are one of the most common causes of healthcare-associated infections.

RESISTANCE OF CONCERN

Resistance to methicillin and related antibiotics (e.g., nafcillin, oxacillin) and resistance to cephalosporins are of concern.

PUBLIC HEALTH THREAT

CDC estimates 80,461 invasive MRSA infections and 11,285 related deaths occurred in 2011. An unknown but much higher number of less severe infections occurred in both the community and in healthcare settings.

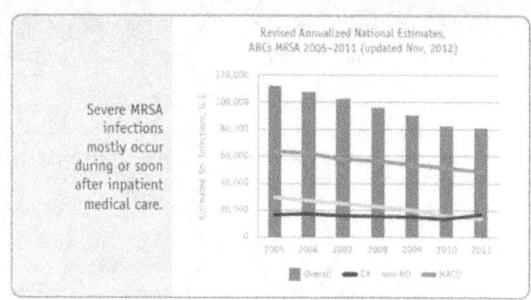

Revised Annualized National Estimates, ABCs MRSA 2005–2011 (updated Nov. 2012)

Severe MRSA infections mostly occur during or soon after inpatient medical care.

For more information about data methods and references, please see technical appendix.

METHICILLIN-RESISTANT STAPHYLOCOCCUS AUREUS (MRSA)

FIGHTING THE SPREAD OF RESISTANCE

Although still a common and severe threat to patients, invasive MRSA infections in healthcare settings appear to be declining. Between 2005 and 2011 overall rates of invasive MRSA dropped 31%; the largest declines (54%) were observed among infections occurring during hospitalization. Success began with preventing central-line associated bloodstream infections with MRSA, where rates fell nearly 50% from 1997 to 2007.

During the past decade, rates of MRSA infections have increased rapidly among the general population (people who have not recently received care in a healthcare setting). There is some evidence that these increases are slowing, but they are not following the same downward trends as healthcare-associated MRSA.

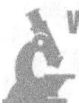

WHAT CDC IS DOING

- Tracking illness and identifying risk factors for drug-resistant infections using two systems, the National Healthcare Safety Network and the Emerging Infections Program.
- Providing states and facilities with outbreak support such as staff expertise, prevention guidelines, tools, and lab assistance.
- Developing tests and prevention recommendations to control drug-resistant infections.
- Helping healthcare facilities improve antibiotic prescribing practices.

WHAT YOU CAN DO

States and Communities Can:

- Know resistance trends in your region.
- Coordinate local and regional infection tracking and control efforts.
- Require facilities to alert each other when transferring patients with any infection.

Healthcare CEOs, Medical Officers, and Other Healthcare Facility Leaders Can:

- Require and strictly enforce CDC guidance for infection detection, prevention, tracking, and reporting.
- Make sure your lab can accurately identify infections and alert clinical and infection prevention staff when these bacteria are present.
- Know infection and resistance trends in your facility and in the facilities around you.
- When transferring a patient, require staff to notify the other facility about all infections.
- Join or start regional infection prevention efforts.
- Promote wise antibiotic use.

Healthcare Providers Can:

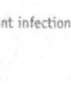

- Know when and types of drug-resistant infections are present in your facility and patients.
- Request immediate alerts when the lab identifies drug-resistant infections in your patients.
- Alert the other facility when you transfer a patient with a drug-resistant infection.
- Protect patients from drug-resistant infections.
- Follow relevant guidelines and precautions at every patient encounter.
- Prescribe antibiotics wisely.
- Remove temporary medical devices such as catheters and ventilators as soon as no longer needed.

Patients and Their Loved Ones Can:

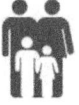

- Ask everyone, including doctors, nurses, other medical staff, and visitors, to wash their hands before touching the patient.
- Take antibiotics only and exactly as prescribed.

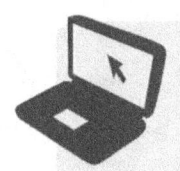

ONLINE RESOURCES

Resources CDC's MRSA website
www.cdc.gov/hai/mrsa

Prevention Guidelines for MRSA
www.cdc.gov/hicpac/pubs.html

Medscape/CDC Expert Commentaries about MRSA
http://www.medscape.com/partners/cdc/public/cdc-commentary

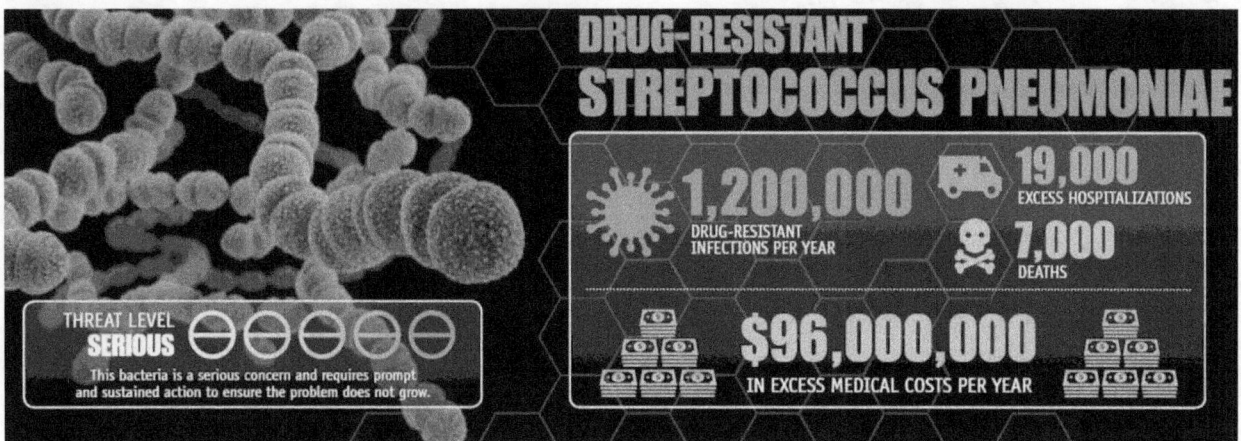

DRUG-RESISTANT
STREPTOCOCCUS PNEUMONIAE

1,200,000 DRUG-RESISTANT INFECTIONS PER YEAR

19,000 EXCESS HOSPITALIZATIONS

7,000 DEATHS

$96,000,000 IN EXCESS MEDICAL COSTS PER YEAR

THREAT LEVEL
SERIOUS
This bacteria is a serious concern and requires prompt and sustained action to ensure the problem does not grow.

Streptococcus pneumoniae (S. pneumoniae, or pneumococcus) is the leading cause of bacterial pneumonia and meningitis in the United States. It also is a major cause of bloodstream infections and ear and sinus infections.

RESISTANCE OF CONCERN

S. pneumoniae has developed resistance to drugs in the penicillin and erythromycin groups. Examples of these drugs include amoxicillin and azithromycin (Zithromax, Z-Pak). *S. pneumoniae* has also developed resistance to less commonly used drugs.

PUBLIC HEALTH THREAT

Pneumococcal disease, whether or not resistant to antibiotics, is a major public health problem. Pneumococcal disease causes 4 million disease episodes and 22,000 deaths annually. Pneumococcal ear infections (otitis media) are the most common type of pneumococcal disease among children, causing 1.5 million infections that often result in antibiotic use. Pneumococcal pneumonia is another important form of pneumococcal disease. Each year, nearly 160,000 children younger than 5 years old see a doctor or are admitted to the hospital with pneumococcal pneumonia. Among adults, over 600,000 seek care for or are hospitalized with pneumococcal pneumonia. Pneumococcal pneumonia accounts for 72% of all direct medical costs for treatment of pneumococcal disease.

In 30% of severe *S. pneumoniae* cases, the bacteria are fully resistant to one or more clinically relevant antibiotics. Resistant infections complicate treatment and can result in almost 1,200,000 illnesses and 7,000 deaths per year. Cases of resistant pneumococcal pneumonia result in about 32,000 additional doctor visits and about 19,000 additional hospitalizations each year. The excess costs associated with these cases are approximately $96 million.

Invasive pneumococcal disease means that bacteria invade parts of the body that are normally sterile, and when this happens, disease is usually severe, causing hospitalization or even death. The majority of cases and deaths occur among adults 50 years or older, with the highest rates among those 65 years or older. Almost everyone who gets invasive pneumococcal disease needs treatment in the hospital.

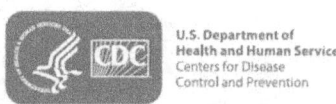

U.S. Department of Health and Human Services
Centers for Disease Control and Prevention

167

DRUG-RESISTANT
STREPTOCOCCUS PNEUMONIAE

FIGHTING THE SPREAD OF RESISTANCE

Pneumococcal conjugate vaccine (PCV) is an effective tool to prevent infections. Vaccine use has not only reduced the burden of invasive pneumococcal disease, but it has also reduced antibiotic resistance by blocking the transmission of resistant *S. pneumoniae* strains. From 2000–2009, PCV7 provided protection against seven pneumococcal strains, and beginning in 2010 use of PCV13 expanded that protection to 13 strains. Achieving high vaccination coverage and encouraging appropriate antibiotic use will slow the spread of pneumococcal resistance. Using the right antibiotic at the right time is crucial.

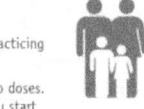

WHAT CDC IS DOING

Through partnerships between CDC, state health departments, and universities, CDC is tracking *S. pneumoniae* through its Active Bacterial Core surveillance (ABCs). CDC is promoting appropriate antibiotic use among outpatient health care providers and the public through its Get Smart: Know When Antibiotics Work program. As part of this program, CDC hosts Get Smart About Antibiotic Week, an annual one week observance of the importance of appropriate antibiotic use and its impact on antibiotic resistance. CDC is also working with many partners in the U.S. to ensure that pneumococcal vaccines are available for children and that uptake is high.

WHAT YOU CAN DO

- Prevent infections by getting recommended vaccines and practicing good hand hygiene.
- Take antibiotics exactly as the doctor prescribes. Do not skip doses. Complete the prescribed course of treatment, even when you start feeling better.
- Only take antibiotics prescribed for you; do not share or use leftover antibiotics.
- Do not save antibiotics for the next illness. Discard any leftover medication once the prescribed course of treatment is completed.
- Do not ask for antibiotics when your doctor thinks you do not need them.

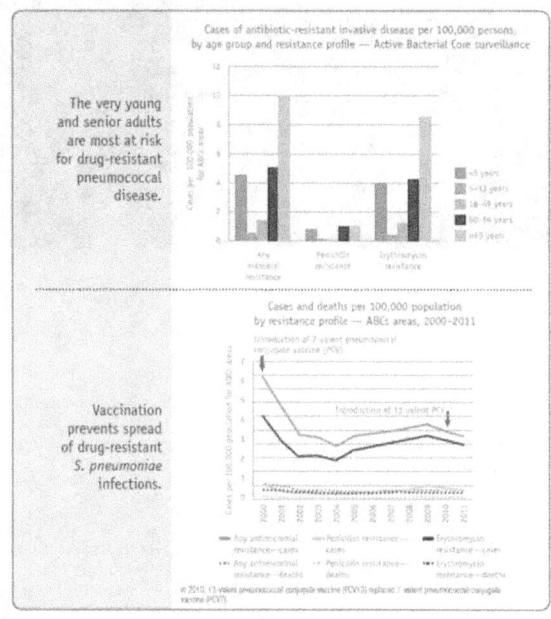

The very young and senior adults are most at risk for drug-resistant pneumococcal disease.

Cases of antibiotic-resistant invasive disease per 100,000 persons, by age group and resistance profile — Active Bacterial Core surveillance

Vaccination prevents spread of drug-resistant *S. pneumoniae* infections.

Cases and deaths per 100,000 population by resistance profile — ABCs areas, 2000–2011

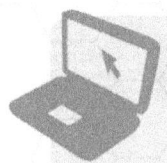

ONLINE RESOURCES

Pneumococcal Disease
www.cdc.gov/pneumococcal

Pneumococcal Vaccine Recommendations
http://www.cdc.gov/vaccines/vpd-vac/pneumo/in-short-both.htm#who

Get Smart: Know When Antibiotics Work Program
http://www.cdc.gov/getsmart/

Active Bacterial Core surveillance (ABCs)
http://www.cdc.gov/abcs/index.html

Drug-Resistant *Streptococcus pneumoniae* (DRSP) Surveillance Toolkit
http://www.cdc.gov/abcs/reports-findings/surv-manual.html

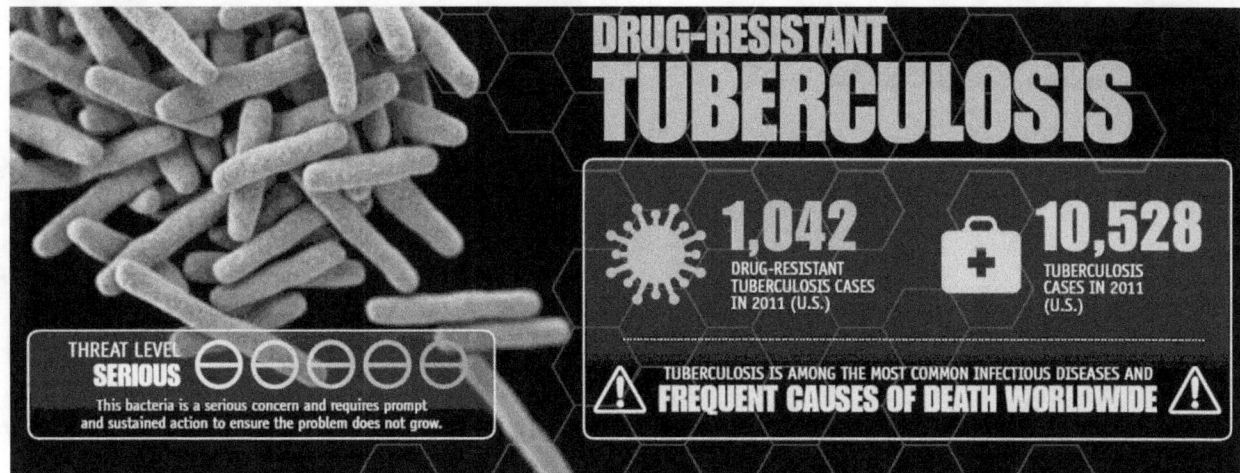

DRUG-RESISTANT
TUBERCULOSIS

1,042
DRUG-RESISTANT
TUBERCULOSIS CASES
IN 2011 (U.S.)

10,528
TUBERCULOSIS
CASES IN 2011
(U.S.)

THREAT LEVEL
SERIOUS
This bacteria is a serious concern and requires prompt
and sustained action to ensure the problem does not grow.

TUBERCULOSIS IS AMONG THE MOST COMMON INFECTIOUS DISEASES AND
FREQUENT CAUSES OF DEATH WORLDWIDE

Tuberculosis (TB) is among the most common infectious diseases and a frequent cause of death worldwide. TB is caused by the bacteria *Mycobacterium tuberculosis* (*M. tuberculosis*) and is spread most commonly through the air. *M. tuberculosis* can affect any part of the body, but disease is found most often in the lungs. In most cases, TB is treatable and curable with the available first-line TB drugs; however, in some cases, *M. tuberculosis* can be resistant to one or more of the drugs used to treat it. Drug-resistant TB is more challenging to treat — it can be complex and requires more time and more expensive drugs that often have more side effects. Extensively Drug-Resistant TB (XDR TB) is resistant to most TB drugs; therefore, patients are left with treatment options that are much less effective. The major factors driving TB drug resistance are incomplete or wrong treatment, short drug supply, and lack of new drugs. In the United States most drug-resistant TB is found among persons born outside of the country.

RESISTANCE OF CONCERN

- Resistance to antibiotics used for standard therapy
- Resistance to isoniazid (INH)
- Some TB is multidrug-resistant (MDR), showing resistance to at least INH and rifampicin (RMP), two essential first-line drugs
- Some TB is XDR TB, defined as MDR TB plus resistance to any fluoroquinolone and to any of the three second-line injectable drugs (i.e., amikacin, kanamycin, capreomycin)

PUBLIC HEALTH THREAT

Of a total of 10,528 cases of TB in the United States reported in 2011, antibiotic resistance was identified in 1,042, or 9.90%, of all TB cases.

	Number of cases	Cases per 100,000 U.S. population	Percent of all TB cases in U.S.
Any first-line resistance	1,042	0.33	10%
INH resistance	740	0.24	7%
MDR TB	124	0.04	1%
XDR TB	6	0.0019	<1%
Deaths caused by antibiotic-resistant TB	50		

For more information about data methods and references, please see technical appendix.

169

DRUG-RESISTANT TUBERCULOSIS

FIGHTING THE SPREAD OF RESISTANCE

Health care providers can help prevent drug-resistant TB by quickly suspecting and diagnosing cases, following recommended treatment guidelines, monitoring patients' response to treatment, and ensuring therapy is completed. Additional drug-resistant TB prevention measures include implementing effective infection control procedures that help limit exposure to known drug-resistant TB patients in settings such as hospitals, prisons, or homeless shelters.

WHAT CDC IS DOING

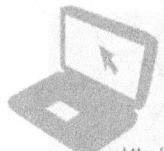

CDC conducts ongoing surveillance for drug-resistant TB in all 50 states and the District of Columbia using the National Tuberculosis Surveillance System (NTSS). The TB Genotyping Information Management System (TBGIMS), a Web-based system designed to improve access and dissemination of genotyping information nationwide, complements the ongoing surveillance for drug- resistant TB by linking genotyping results to surveillance data. In 2009, CDC implemented the Molecular Detection of Drug Resistance Service (MDDR), a national clinical referral service which provides rapid confirmation of MDR and XDR TB. Molecular drug-resistant testing enhances but does not replace culture or conventional drug-susceptibility testing.

Other CDC activities directed at preventing spread of drug-resistant TB include funding of five TB Regional Training and Medical Consultation Centers (RTMCCs) from 2013–2017. The RTMCCs are regionally assigned to cover all 50 states and the U.S. territories. One of the primary purposes of each RTMCC is to provide medical consultation to TB programs and medical providers, particularly for complex, drug-resistant cases. Additionally, the RTMCCs offer trainings that provide information on diagnosing and treating drug-resistant TB.

Additionally, CDC international activities include studies to improve first and second line antibiotic use in patients with drug-resistant TB.

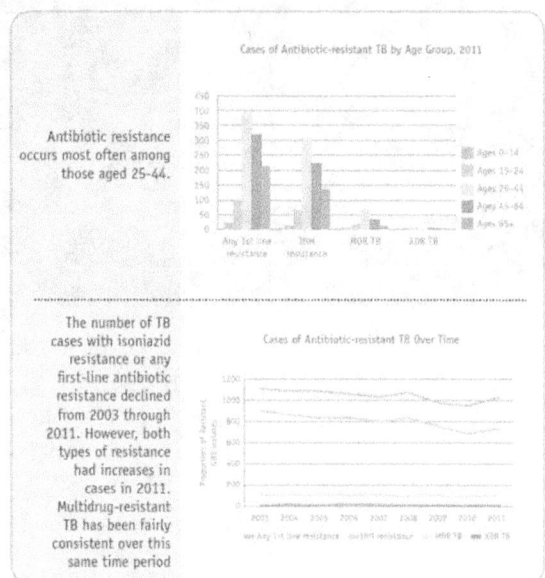

Antibiotic resistance occurs most often among those aged 25-44.

Cases of Antibiotic-resistant TB by Age Group, 2011

The number of TB cases with isoniazid resistance or any first-line antibiotic resistance declined from 2003 through 2011. However, both types of resistance had increases in cases in 2011. Multidrug-resistant TB has been fairly consistent over this same time period

Cases of Antibiotic-resistant TB Over Time

ONLINE RESOURCES

http://www.cdc.gov/tb/

http://www.cdc.gov/tb/topic/drtb/default.htm

http://www.cdc.gov/tb/publications/factsheets/drtb/mdrtb.htm

http://www.cdc.gov/tb/topic/drtb/xdrtb.htm

http://www.cdc.gov/tb/statistics/reports/2011/default.htm

http://www.cdc.gov/tb/topic/Laboratory/mddr.htm

http://www.aphl.org/aphlprograms/infectious/tuberculosis/Pages/default.aspx

http://www.tbcontrollers.org/

http://www.who.int/tb/publications/mdr_surveillance/en/index.html

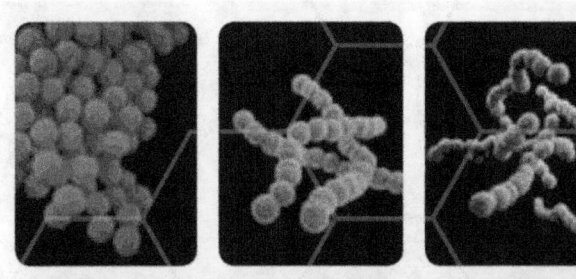

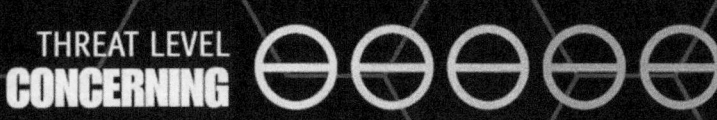

THREAT LEVEL
CONCERNING ⊖ ⊖ ⊖ ⊖ ⊖   These bacteria are concerning, and careful monitoring and prevention action are needed.

MICROORGANISMS WITH A THREAT LEVEL OF CONCERNING

Vancomycin-resistant *Staphylococcus aureus* (VRSA)

Erythromycin-resistant **Group A** *Streptococcus*

Clindamycin-resistant **Group B** *Streptococcus*

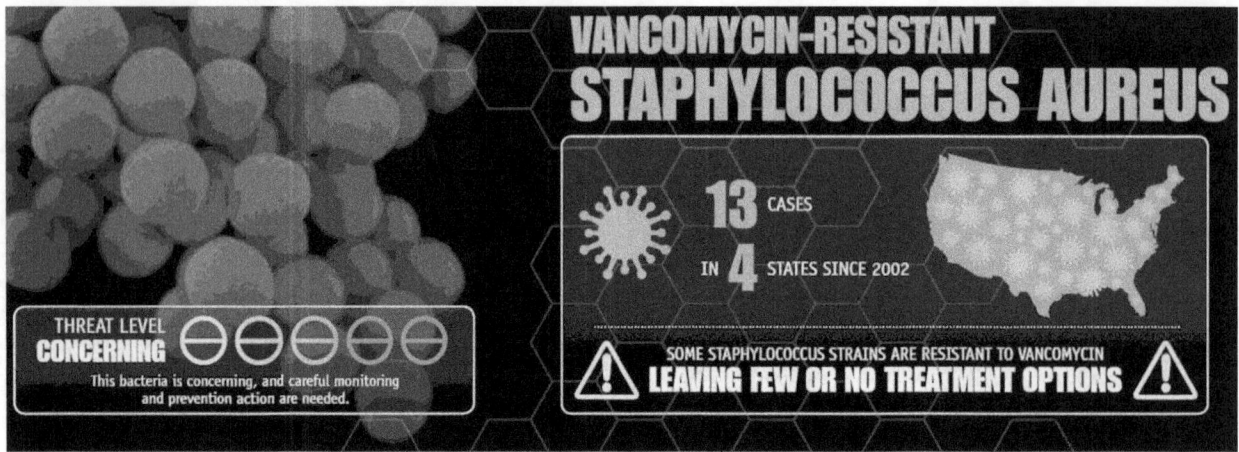

VANCOMYCIN-RESISTANT
STAPHYLOCOCCUS AUREUS

13 CASES

IN **4** STATES SINCE 2002

THREAT LEVEL
CONCERNING ⊖⊖⊖⊖⊖
This bacteria is concerning, and careful monitoring
and prevention action are needed.

SOME STAPHYLOCOCCUS STRAINS ARE RESISTANT TO VANCOMYCIN
⚠ **LEAVING FEW OR NO TREATMENT OPTIONS** ⚠

Staphylococcus aureus is a common type of bacteria that is found on the skin. During medical procedures when patients require catheters or ventilators or undergo surgical procedures, *Staphylococcus aureus* can enter the body and cause infections. When *Staphylococcus aureus* becomes resistant to vancomycin, there are few treatment options available because vancomycin-resistant *S. aureus* bacteria identified to date were also resistant to methicillin and other classes of antibiotics.

RESISTANCE OF CONCERN

In rare cases, CDC has identified *Staphylococcus aureus* that is resistant to vancomycin, the antibiotic most frequently used to treat serious *S. aureus* infections.

PUBLIC HEALTH THREAT

A total of 13 cases of vancomycin-resistant *Staphylococcus aureus* (VRSA) have been identified in the United States since 2002.

VRSA infection continues to be a rare occurrence. A few existing factors seem to predispose case patients to VRSA infection, including:

- Prior MRSA and enterococcal infections or colonization
- Underlying conditions (such as chronic skin ulcers and diabetes)
- Previous treatment with vancomycin

	Number of cases	Cases per 100,000 U.S. population	Percentage of all *Genus* species cases in U.S.	Number of deaths	Deaths per 100,000 U.S. population
Vancomycin-resistant *Staphylococcus aureus*	13	N/A	N/A	0	N/A

For more information about data methods and references, please see technical appendix.

172

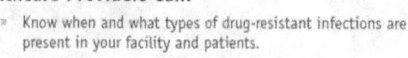
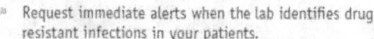

FIGHTING THE SPREAD OF RESISTANCE

WHAT CDC IS DOING

- Confirming cases after being notified by local public health authorities.
- Providing states and facilities with outbreak support such as staff expertise, prevention guidelines, tools, and lab assistance.
- Developing tests and prevention recommendations to control drug-resistant infections.
- Helping medical facilities improve antibiotic prescribing practices.

WHAT YOU CAN DO

States and Communities Can:

- Know resistance trends in your region.
- Coordinate local and regional infection tracking and control efforts.
- Require facilities to alert each other when transferring patients with any infection.

Healthcare CEOs, Medical Officers, and Other Healthcare Facility Leaders Can:

- Require and strictly enforce CDC guidance for infection detection, prevention, tracking, and reporting.
- Make sure your lab can accurately identify infections, and alert clinical and infection prevention staff when these bacteria are present.
- Know infection and resistance trends in your facility and in the facilities around you.
- When transferring a patient, require staff to notify the other facility about all infections.
- Join or start regional infection prevention efforts.
- Promote wise antibiotic use.

Healthcare Providers Can:

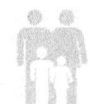

- Know when and what types of drug-resistant infections are present in your facility and patients.
- Request immediate alerts when the lab identifies drug-resistant infections in your patients.
- Alert the other facility when you transfer a patient with a drug-resistant infection.
- Treat wounds aggressively.
- Use vancomycin responsibly.
- Protect patients from drug-resistant infections.
  - Follow relevant guidelines and precautions at every patient encounter.
  - Prescribe antibiotics wisely.
  - Remove temporary medical devices such as catheters and ventilators as soon as no longer needed.

Patients and Their Loved Ones Can:

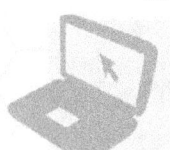

- Ask everyone, including doctors, nurses, other medical staff, and visitors, to wash their hands before touching the patient.
- Take antibiotics only and exactly as prescribed.

ONLINE RESOURCES

Vancomycin-Intermediate/Resistant Staphylococcus (VISA/VRSA) in Healthcare Settings
http://www.cdc.gov/HAI/organisms/visa_vrsa/visa_vrsa.html

Healthcare-associated Infections (HAIs), Guidelines and Recommendations
www.cdc.gov/hicpac/pubs.html

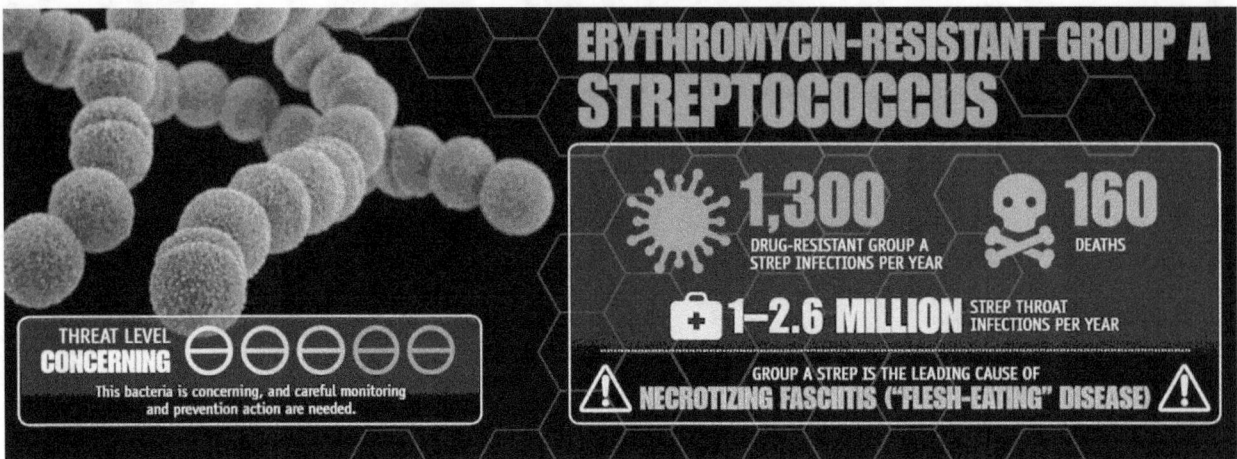

ERYTHROMYCIN-RESISTANT GROUP A
STREPTOCOCCUS

1,300 DRUG-RESISTANT GROUP A STREP INFECTIONS PER YEAR

160 DEATHS

1–2.6 MILLION STREP THROAT INFECTIONS PER YEAR

GROUP A STREP IS THE LEADING CAUSE OF
NECROTIZING FASCIITIS ("FLESH-EATING" DISEASE)

Group A *Streptococcus* (GAS) causes many illnesses, including pharyngitis (strep throat), streptococcal toxic shock syndrome, necrotizing fasciitis ("flesh-eating" disease), scarlet fever, rheumatic fever, and skin infections such as impetigo.

RESISTANCE OF CONCERN

GAS has developed resistance to clindamycin and a category of drugs called macrolides. Macrolides include erythromycin, azithromycin and clarithromycin. GAS has also developed resistance to a less commonly used drug—tetracycline. Of these, resistance to erythromycin and the other macrolide antibiotics is of the most immediate concern.

PUBLIC HEALTH THREAT

Each year in the United States, erythromycin-resistant, invasive GAS causes 1,300 illnesses and 160 deaths.

GAS is a leading cause of upper respiratory tract infections such as strep throat. There are 1-2.6 million cases of strep throat in the U.S. each year. These bacteria are also the leading cause of necrotizing fasciitis, an invasive disease that can be fatal in 25%-35% of cases. Invasive disease means that bacteria invade parts of the body that are normally sterile. When this happens, disease is usually very severe, causing hospitalization or even death. Those at highest risk for invasive disease are the elderly, those with skin lesions, young children, people in group living situations such as nursing homes, and those with underlying medical conditions, such as diabetes.

Penicillin is the recommended first-line treatment for GAS infections. Amoxicillin is a type of penicillin that is often used to treat strep throat. Currently, GAS is not resistant to treatment with penicillin. If resistance to penicillin emerges, it would severely compromise treatment of invasive GAS infections. For people who are allergic to penicillin, two of the alternative antibiotics, azithromycin and clarithromycin, can be used to treat strep throat. In fact, azithromycin is prescribed more commonly than penicillin. Of GAS bacterial samples tested at CDC from 2010 and 2011, 10% were erythromycin-resistant (and therefore resistant to other macrolides such as azithromycin and clarithromycin), while 3.4% were clindamycin-resistant. Increasing resistance to erythromycin will complicate treatment of strep throat, particularly for those who cannot tolerate penicillin.

A more current concern is the increase in bacteria that show the genetic potential for becoming resistant to clindamycin. Clindamycin has a unique role in treatment of severe GAS infections. For severe, life-threatening infections, like necrotizing fasciitis and toxic shock syndrome, a combination of penicillin and clindamycin is recommended for treatment.

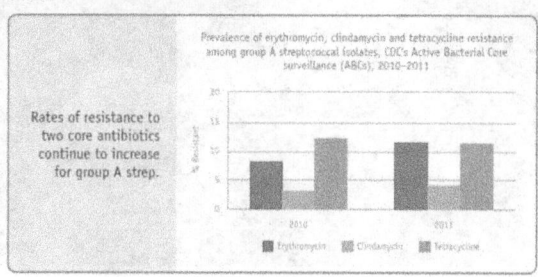

FIGHTING THE SPREAD OF RESISTANCE

Encouraging appropriate antibiotic use, including using the right antibiotic at the right time, and for the right amount of time, is crucial to preventing the spread of drug-resistant GAS. Doctors should adhere to the recommended antibiotics for treating GAS infections, including using penicillin or amoxicillin whenever possible.

WHAT CDC IS DOING

CDC has collaborated with the Infectious Diseases Society of America to update guidance on diagnosing strep throat and selecting antibiotics to treat it. These guidelines reinforce appropriate use of antibiotics for this common illness. CDC is also promoting appropriate antibiotic use among outpatient healthcare providers and the public through its Get Smart: Know When Antibiotics Work program. As part of this program, CDC hosts Get Smart About Antibiotics Week, an annual one-week observance of the importance of appropriate antibiotic use and its impact on antibiotic resistance. Through partnerships between CDC, state health departments, and universities, CDC is tracking GAS through Active Bacterial Core surveillance (ABCs).

WHAT YOU CAN DO

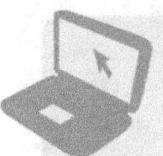

- Prevent infections by practicing good hand hygiene.
- Take antibiotics exactly as the doctor prescribes. Do not skip doses. Complete the prescribed course of treatment, even when you start feeling better.
- Only take antibiotics prescribed for you. Do not share or use leftover antibiotics.
- Do not save antibiotics for the next illness. Discard any leftover medication once the prescribed course of treatment is completed.
- Do not ask for antibiotics when your doctor thinks you do not need them.

Prevalence of erythromycin, clindamycin and tetracycline resistance among group A streptococcal isolates, CDC's Active Bacterial Core surveillance (ABCs), 2010–2011

Rates of resistance to two core antibiotics continue to increase for group A strep.

2010   2011

■ Erythromycin   ■ Clindamycin   ■ Tetracycline

ONLINE RESOURCES

Active Bacterial Core surveillance (ABCs)
http://www.cdc.gov/abcs/index.html

Get Smart: Know When Antibiotics Work Program
http://www.cdc.gov/getsmart/

Group A Strep
http://www.cdc.gov/ncidod/dbmd/diseaseinfo/groupastreptococcal_g.htm

Necrotizing Fasciitis
http://www.cdc.gov/features/necrotizingfasciitis/

Strep Throat
http://www.cdc.gov/features/strepthroat/

Scarlet Fever
http://www.cdc.gov/features/scarletfever/

175

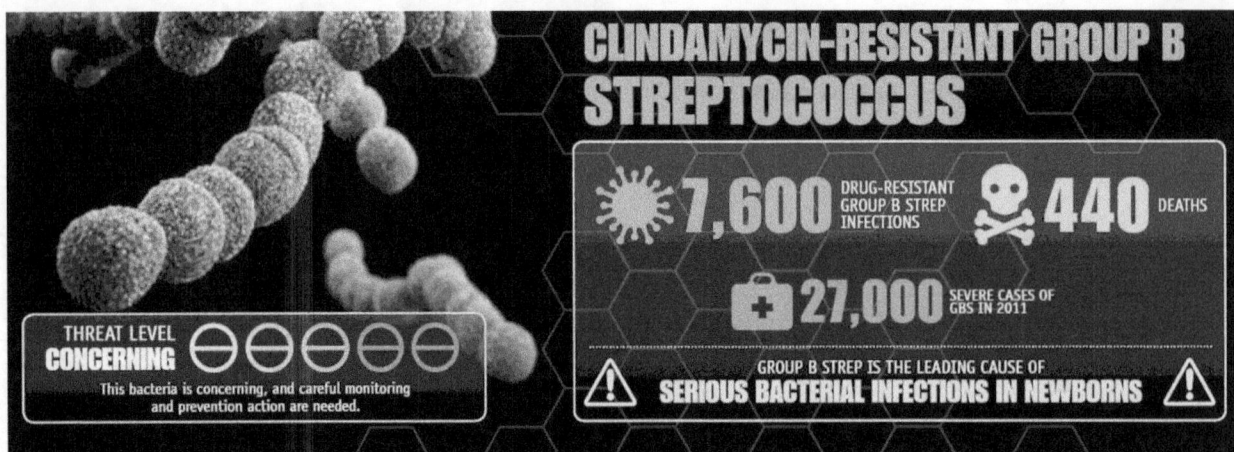

Group B *Streptococcus* (GBS) is a type of bacteria that can cause severe illnesses in people of all ages, ranging from bloodstream infections (sepsis) and pneumonia to meningitis and skin infections.

RESISTANCE OF CONCERN

GBS has developed resistance to clindamycin and erythromycin. GBS that are resistant to erythromycin will also be resistant to azithromycin. Recently, the very first cases with resistance to vancomycin have been detected among adults. These cases are extremely rare and also very concerning since vancomycin is the most commonly used drug for treatment of potentially resistant gram-positive infections in adults. Strains with decreasing responsiveness to treatment with penicillin drugs have been described but remain very rare. Resistance to clindamycin is of the most immediate clinical concern, although the other forms of resistance are worrisome.

PUBLIC HEALTH THREAT

Each year in the United States, clindamycin-resistant Group B Strep causes an estimated 7,600 illnesses and 440 deaths.

In the United States, GBS is the leading cause of serious bacterial infections in newborns, including bloodstream infections, meningitis, and pneumonia. When these GBS infections occur in the first 7 days of life, they are known as early-onset disease. To prevent early-onset disease in newborns, antibiotics are given during labor and delivery to mothers who test positive for GBS (tested at 35–37 weeks of pregnancy with a vaginal/rectal swab) and to those who have other risk factors for passing GBS to their newborns.

GBS also is one of the most common causes of meningitis and other severe infections in infants from 7 days to 3 months old (late-onset disease). GBS is also an increasing cause of bloodstream infections, pneumonia, skin and soft tissue infections, and bone and joint infections in adults, especially among pregnant women, the elderly, and people with certain medical conditions such as diabetes.

CDC estimates from preliminary data that 27,000 cases of severe GBS disease, such as blood infections or meningitis, occurred in 2011, causing 1,575 deaths. Forty-nine percent of GBS isolates (samples) tested were erythromycin-resistant, and 28% were clindamycin-resistant. Although the incidence of early-onset disease has been decreasing, the proportion of GBS infections resistant to erythromycin and clindamycin has increased steadily since 2000.

Resistance to the penicillin drug class could threaten the success of strategies to prevent early-onset disease and lead to treatment failures since penicillin drugs are the top choice for treating GBS. Additionally, the increasing resistance to recommended second-line drugs, clindamycin and erythromycin, limits prevention and treatment for patients with GBS who are allergic to penicillin.

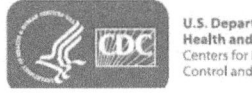

U.S. Department of Health and Human Services
Centers for Disease Control and Prevention

FIGHTING THE SPREAD OF RESISTANCE

Doctors should test all pregnant women for GBS at 35–37 weeks of pregnancy and adhere to the recommended antibiotics during labor and delivery for prevention of early-onset disease. Broad efforts to promote appropriate use of antibiotics in outpatient and inpatient settings will also help minimize the spread of resistance among GBS bacteria.

WHAT CDC IS DOING

CDC, in collaboration with professional associations, has developed evidence-based Guidelines for the Prevention of Perinatal Group B Streptococcal Disease. These guidelines discuss diagnosis and management, and recommendations are provided regarding antibiotic choices and dosing. They also support GBS screening for all pregnant women at 35–37 weeks of pregnancy and use of antibiotics during labor and delivery to prevent newborn infection. Through partnerships between CDC, state health departments, and universities, CDC is tracking GBS through its Active Bacterial Core surveillance (ABCs). This program monitors antibiotic resistance and has contributed to the detection of the very first cases in the U.S. of vancomycin-resistant GBS, as well as tracking of susceptibility trends of other antibiotics important for treatment of GBS. CDC is promoting appropriate antibiotic use among outpatient health care providers and the public through its Get Smart: Know When Antibiotics Work program.

WHAT YOU CAN DO

- Pregnant women should talk to their doctor or nurse about their GBS status and let them know of any medication allergies during a checkup.

- When women get to the hospital or birthing center for delivery, they should remind their doctor or nurse if they have GBS and if they are allergic to any medications.

- Practice appropriate antibiotic use whenever you see a doctor or are prescribed an antibiotic for any condition:

  - Take antibiotics exactly as the doctor prescribes. Do not skip doses. Complete the prescribed course of treatment, even when you start feeling better.

  - Only take antibiotics prescribed for you. Do not share or use leftover antibiotics.

  - Do not save antibiotics for the next illness. Discard any leftover medication once the prescribed course of treatment is completed.

  - Do not ask for antibiotics when your doctor thinks you do not need them.

Group B strep continues to become more resistant to two major antibiotics, leaving those allergic to first line drugs in jeopardy.

Proportion of Group B *Streptococcus* isolates resistant to erythromycin and clindamycin—
Active Bacterial Core surveillance (ABCs), 2000-2010*

*Most recent data available

Early-onset group B strep disease has declined by 80% since the introduction of evidence-based prevention strategies.

Incidence of Early-Onset Disease Caused by Group B *Streptococcus*—
Active Bacterial Core surveillance (ABCs), 1989-2010

ACOG = American College of Obstetricians and Gynecologists, AAP = American Academy of Pediatrics

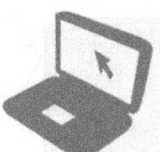

ONLINE RESOURCES

Group B Strep (GBS)
http://www.cdc.gov/groupbstrep/about/index.html

Active Bacterial Core surveillance (ABCs)
http://www.cdc.gov/abcs/index.html

Technical Appendix

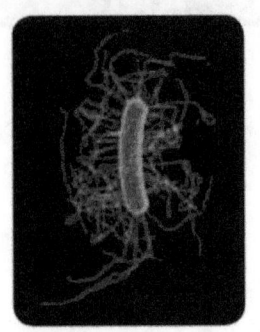

Technical Appendix

Clostridium difficile

Methods

National estimates of the number of *Clostridium difficile (C. difficile)* infections (CDI) requiring hospitalization or in already hospitalized patients were obtained from the data submitted through the Emerging Infections Program's *C. difficile* surveillance in 2011, of 34 counties in 10 U.S. states (http://www.cdc.gov/hai/eip/cdiff_techinfo.html). During 2011, a total of 15,452 CDI cases were identified across the participating sites. Data on hospitalization following CDI or at the time of infection were obtained for all cases from 8 of 10 U.S. states and from a random sample of 33% from cases from the other 2 states. The sampled cases were used to estimate total number of hospitalizations in the 2 states where sampling was performed. The national estimates were made using 2011 population estimates from U.S. Census Bureau adjusting for age, gender and race distribution of the American population.[1] Approximately 18% of cases were reported without a race value. Multiple imputation was used to estimate the missing race based on the data that are available and the results were summarized. The *C. difficile* attributable mortality was estimated from death certificate data.[2] Trends on deaths related to *C. difficile* were obtained from the CDC's National Center for Health Statistics.[3] Estimates were rounded to two significant digits.

References

1   Lessa FC, Mu, Y, Cohen J, Dumyati G, Farley MM, Winston L, Kast K, Holzbauer S, Meek J, Beldavs S, McDonald LC, Fridkin SK. Presented at the IDWeek 2012, Annual Meeting of the Infectious Disease Society of America, Society for Healthcare Epidemiology, Pediatric Infectious Disease Society, and HIV Medical Association; San Diego, October 2012.

2   Hall AJ, Curns AT, McDonald LC, Parashar UD, Lopman BA. The Roles of *Clostridium difficile* and Norovirus Among Gastroenteritis-Associated Deaths in the United States, 1999-2007. Clin Infect Dis. 2012 Jul;55(2):216–23.

3   Kochanek KD, Xu J, Murphy SL, Miniño AM, Kung HC. Deaths: Preliminary Data for 2009. National Vital Statistics Report.

Technical Appendix

Carbapenem-Resistant Enterobacteriaceae

Multidrug-Resistant *Acinetobacter*

Fluconazole-Resistant *Candida*

Extended Spectrum B-lactamase producing
Enterobacteriaceae (ESBLs)

Vancomycin-Resistant *Enterococcus* (VRE)

Multidrug-Resistant *Pseudomonas aeruginosa*

Methods

National estimates of the number of healthcare-associated infections (HAIs) with Enterobacteriaceae, *Pseudomonas aeruginosa*, *Candida*, *Acinetobacter,* or Enterococci were obtained from a 2011 survey of 11,282 patients in 183 hospitals in 10 different states, among whom 452 were identified with at least one HAI for a total of 504 HAIs (some patients had >1 HAI).

Many assumptions were made in deriving national estimates, using these 452 patients, and adjusting for age and length of stay using the 2010 Nationwide Inpatient Sample (NIS), Healthcare Cost and Utilization Project (HCUP), Agency for Healthcare Research and Quality. For 2011, an estimated 647,985 patients had at least one HAI, resulting in an estimated 721,854 HAIs.[1] 481 pathogens were reported among the 504 HAIs detected; 50 *K. pneumonia* or *K. oxytoca* (9.9%), 47 *E. coli* (9.3%), 46 *Enterococci spp.* (9.1%), 36 *P. aeruginosa* (7.1%), 34 *Candida spp.* (6.7%), 8 *Acinetobacter spp.* (1.6%). For each pathogen, the pathogen-specific annual estimate was obtained by multiplying this proportion (of all HAIs) by the national HAI estimate (721,854). Next, the estimated no. of resistant infections was obtained by multiplying the respective pathogen-specific national estimate by the proportion of pathogens reported as non-susceptible to the antimicrobial of interest from other CDC data systems. For Enterobacteriaceae, *Pseudomonas aeruginosa*, *Acinetobacter,* and Enterococci this was CDC's National Healthcare Safety Network and includes the mean percent non-susceptible across the device and procedure-associated HAIs reported during 2009–2010[2]; see individual fact sheets in this report for percent resistance for each pathogen.

For *Candida* by the proportion of *Candida* species testing non-susceptible to fluconazole that were submitted to CDC for confirmatory testing as part of the Emerging Infections Program Surveillance of *Candida* bloodstream infections during 2008-2011.[3] In this program a total of 2,675 *Candida* species isolates associated with bloodstream infections were submitted as part of the EIP population-based surveillance in 2 US cities, azole resistance was identified in 165 cases, or 7%.

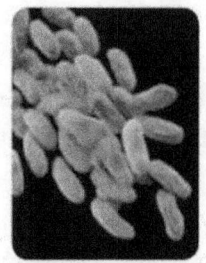
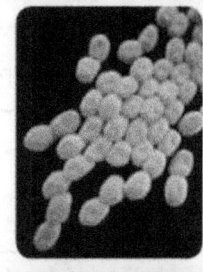
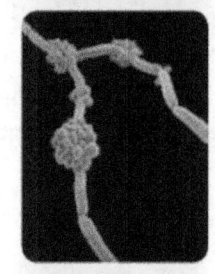
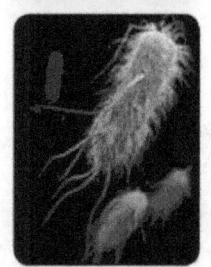
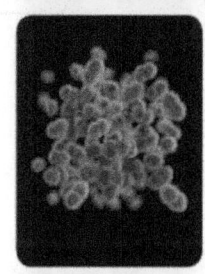
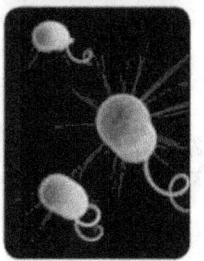

The number of deaths attributable to the antimicrobial-resistant healthcare-associated infection was determined by multiplying the estimated number of resistant infections by 6.5%, an overall estimate of attributable mortality from antibiotic-resistant hospital-onset infections previously determined.[4] This estimate accounts for the overall distribution of the different types of infections commonly caused by antibiotic-resistant pathogens in hospitalized patients and is generally much lower than the crude mortality observed in many of these patients owing to their severe underlying disease status. Definitions of multidrug resistance used in this analysis are published elsewhere.[2] The proportion of U.S. hospitals reporting carbapenem-resistant Enterobacteriaceae was derived as reported elsewhere.[5] Estimates were rounded to two significant digits.

References

1   Magill SS, Edwards JR, Bamberg W, Beldavs Z, Dumyati G, Kainer M, Lynfield R, Maloney M, McAllister-Hollod L, Nadle J, Ray SR, Thompson DL, Wilson LE, Fridkin SK. Presented at the IDWeek 2012, Annual Meeting of the Infectious Disease Society of America, Society for Healthcare Epidemiology, Pediatric Infectious Disease Society, and HIV Medical Association; San Diego, October 2012.

2   Sievert DM, Ricks P, Edwards JR, Schneider A, Patel J, Srinivasan A, Kallen A, Limbago B, Fridkin S; National Healthcare Safety Network (NHSN) Team and Participating NHSN Facilities. Antimicrobial-resistant pathogens associated with healthcare-associated infections: summary of data reported to the National Healthcare Safety Network at the Centers for Disease Control and Prevention, 2009–2010. Infect Control Hosp Epidemiol. 2013 Jan;34(1):1–14

3   Cleveland AA, Farley MM, Harrison LH, Stein B, Hollick R, Lockhart SR, Magill SS, Derado G, Park BJ, Chiller TM. Changes in incidence and antifungal drug resistance in candidemia: results from population-based laboratory surveillance in Atlanta and Baltimore, 2008–2011. Clin Infect Dis. 2012 Nov 15;55(10):1352–61.

4   Roberts RR, Hota B, Ahmad I, Scott RD 2nd, Foster SD, Abbasi F, Schabowski S, Kampe LM, Ciavarella GG, Supino M, Naples J, Cordell R, Levy SB, Weinstein RA. Hospital and societal costs of antimicrobial-resistant infections in a Chicago teaching hospital: implications for antibiotic stewardship. Clin Infect Dis. 2009 Oct 15;49(8):1175–84

5   Centers for Disease Control and Prevention (CDC). Vital Signs: Carbapenem-resistant Enterobacteriaceae. MMWR Morb Mortal Wkly Rep. 2013 Mar 8;62(9):165–70.

Technical Appendix

Neisseria gonorrhoeae

Methods

Estimates of the number of gonococcal infections with any resistance pattern, reduced susceptibility to cephalosporins or azithromycin, or resistance to tetracycline are reported. They are derived by multiplying an estimate of the annual number of gonococcal infections in the United States[1] by the prevalence of reduced susceptibility or resistance among urethral *Neisseria gonorrhoeae* isolates collected and tested by the Gonococcal Isolate Surveillance Project (GISP) during 2011.[2]

Many assumptions were made in deriving the estimates. Data from the National Health and Nutrition Examination Survey (NHANES) provided accurate gonorrhea prevalence estimates, although NHANES only measures urogenital infections and does not include oropharyngeal or rectal infections. The average duration of infection, used to calculate incidence, was based on expert opinion, due to an absence of published data. Also, estimates of resistance in GISP are nationally representative. However, compared to the regional distribution of reported gonococcal infections, GISP relatively over-samples patients from the West Coast, where resistance has traditionally first emerged in the United States. The Clinical Laboratory Standards Institute categorizes susceptibility to cefixime and ceftriaxone as minimum inhibitory concentrations (MICs) $\leq$0.25 µg/ml.[3] For this analysis, isolates with cefixime MICs $\geq$0.25 µg/ml were considered to have reduced cefixime susceptibility, and isolates with ceftriaxone MICs $\geq$0.125 µg/ml were considered to have reduced ceftriaxone susceptibility. An azithromycin MIC $\geq$2.0 µg/ml was considered to have reduced azithromycin susceptibility, and a tetracycline MIC $\geq$2.0 µg/ml was considered resistant. Resistance to any antimicrobial includes resistance to penicillin (MIC $\geq$ 2 µg/ml), tetracycline, ciprofloxacin (MIC $\geq$ 1µg/ml), or spectinomycin (MIC $\geq$ 128 µg/ml), or reduced susceptibility to the cephalosporins or azithromycin.

GISP, established in 1986, is a sentinel surveillance system with partners that include CDC, sexually transmitted disease clinics at 25–30 sentinel sites, and 5 regional laboratories in the United States.[4] Gonococcal isolates are collected from up to the first 25 men diagnosed with gonococcal urethritis at each sentinel site each month. Antimicrobial susceptibility testing is performed using agar dilution for a panel of antimicrobials that includes penicillin, tetracycline, ciprofloxacin, spectinomycin, cefixime, ceftriaxone, and azithromycin.

References

1   Satterwhite CL et al. Sexually transmitted infections among US women and men: prevalence and incidence estimates, 2008. Sex Transm Dis 2013;40(3):187–93.

2   CDC. Sexually transmitted diseases surveillance 2011. Atlanta: U.S. Department of Health and Human Services; 2012.

3   Clinical and Laboratory Standards Institute. Performance Standards for Antimicrobial Susceptibility Testing; Twenty-Third Informational Supplement. CLSI document M100-S23. Wayne, PA; Clinical and Laboratory Standards Institute; 2013; 33(1):100–102.

4   CDC GISP website: http://www.cdc.gov/std/GISP.

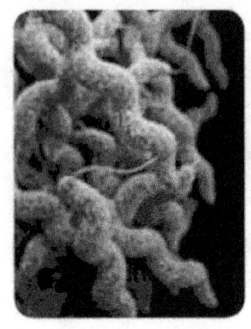

Drug-Resistant *Campylobacter*

Methods

Estimates of the number of illnesses and deaths from infections with *Campylobacter* resistant to ciprofloxacin or azithromycin are reported. They were derived by multiplying an estimate of the annual number of *Campylobacter* illnesses or deaths in the United States[1] by the average prevalence of resistance among *Campylobacter* tested by the National Antimicrobial Resistance Monitoring System (NARMS) during the years 2009–2011. Resistance breakpoints from the NARMS 2011 Human Isolates Report were used.[2]

Many assumptions were made in deriving the estimates. The estimated number of illnesses from resistant *Campylobacter* was divided by the U.S. population and multiplied by 100,000 to calculate the estimated number of illnesses from resistant infections per 100,000 people. The U.S. population in 2006 (approximately 299 million people) was used for the calculations because the estimated number of *Campylobacter* illnesses in the United States was based on this population.[1] The sentinel county survey data displayed in Figure 1 was previously reported.[3]

References

1   Scallan E, Hoekstra RM, Angulo FJ, et al. Foodborne illness acquired in the United States—major pathogens. Emerg Infect Dis 2011;17:7–15.

2   CDC. National Antimicrobial Resistance Monitoring System for Enteric Bacteria (NARMS): Human Isolates Final Report, 2011. Atlanta, Georgia: U.S. Department of Health and Human Services, CDC, 2013.

3   Gupta A, Nelson JM, Barrett TJ, et al. Antimicrobial Resistance among *Campylobacter* Strains, United States, 1997–2001. Emerg Infect Dis 2004;10:1102-9.

Technical Appendix

Drug-Resistant Non-Typhoidal *Salmonella*

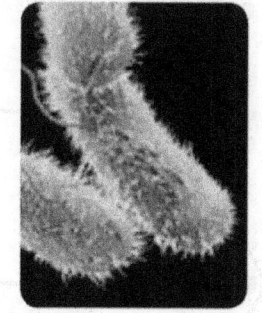

Methods

Estimates of the number of illnesses and deaths from infections with non-typhoidal *Salmonella* resistant to ceftriaxone, resistant or partially resistant to ciprofloxacin, or resistant to five or more antibiotic classes are reported. They were derived by multiplying an estimate of the annual number of non-typhoidal *Salmonella* illnesses or deaths in the United States[1] by the average prevalence of resistance among non-typhoidal *Salmonella* isolates tested by the National Antimicrobial Resistance Monitoring System (NARMS) during the years 2009–2011. Resistance breakpoints from the NARMS 2011 Human Isolates Report were used.[3] For ciprofloxacin, isolates with intermediate susceptibility results (minimum inhibitory concentration of 0.12–0.5 µg/ml) were considered partially resistant.

Many assumptions were made in deriving the estimates. The estimated number of illnesses from resistant *Salmonella* was divided by the U.S. population and multiplied by 100,000 to calculate the estimated number of illnesses from resistant *Salmonella* per 100,000 population. The U.S. population in 2006 (approximately 299 million people) was used for the calculations because the estimated number of non-typhoidal *Salmonella* illnesses in the United States was based on this population.[1] The methods used to estimate the direct medical costs for *Salmonella* infections were previously reported.[2]

References

1 Scallan E, Hoekstra RM, Angulo FJ, et al. Foodborne illness acquired in the United States—major pathogens. Emerg Infect Dis. 2011;17:7–15.

2 CDC. National Antimicrobial Resistance Monitoring System for Enteric Bacteria (NARMS): Human Isolates Final Report, 2011. Atlanta, Georgia: U.S. Department of Health and Human Services, CDC, 2013.

3 CDC. Vital Signs: Incidence and Trends of Infection with Pathogens Transmitted Commonly Through Food—Foodborne Diseases Active Surveillance Network, 10 U.S. Sites, 1996–2010. MMWR 2011;60:749–55.

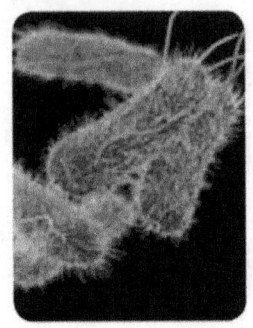

Methods

An estimate of the number of illnesses and deaths from *Salmonella* serotype Typhi resistant or partially resistant to ciprofloxacin was derived by multiplying an estimate of the annual number of illnesses or deaths from typhoid fever in the United States[1] by the average prevalence of ciprofloxacin resistance or partial resistance among *Salmonella* Typhi isolates tested by the National Antimicrobial Resistance Monitoring System (NARMS) during 2009–2011. Resistance breakpoints from the NARMS 2011 Human Isolates Report were used.[2] For ciprofloxacin, isolates with intermediate susceptibility results (minimum inhibitory concentration of 0.12–0.5 µg/ml) were considered partially resistant.

Many assumptions were made in deriving the estimates. The estimated number of illnesses from ciprofloxacin resistant or partially resistant *Salmonella* Typhi was divided by the U.S. population and multiplied by 100,000 to calculate the estimated number of illnesses from resistant or partially resistant infections per 100,000 people. The U.S. population in 2006 (approximately 299 million people) was used for the calculations because the estimated number of typhoid fever illnesses in the United States was based on this population. Worldwide case estimates[3] and pre-antibiotic era mortality[4] are from published sources.

References

1   Scallan E, Hoekstra RM, Angulo FJ, et al. Foodborne illness acquired in the United States—major pathogens. Emerg Infect Dis 2011;17(1):7–15.

2   CDC. National Antimicrobial Resistance Monitoring System for Enteric Bacteria (NARMS): Human Isolates Final Report, 2011. Atlanta, Georgia: U.S. Department of Health and Human Services, CDC, 2013.

3   Crump JA, Mintz ED. Global trends in typhoid and paratyphoid fever. Clin Infect Dis 2010;50(2):241-6.Heymann DL, editor. Control of Communicable Diseases Manual. 19th ed. Washington DC: American Public Health Association; 2008.

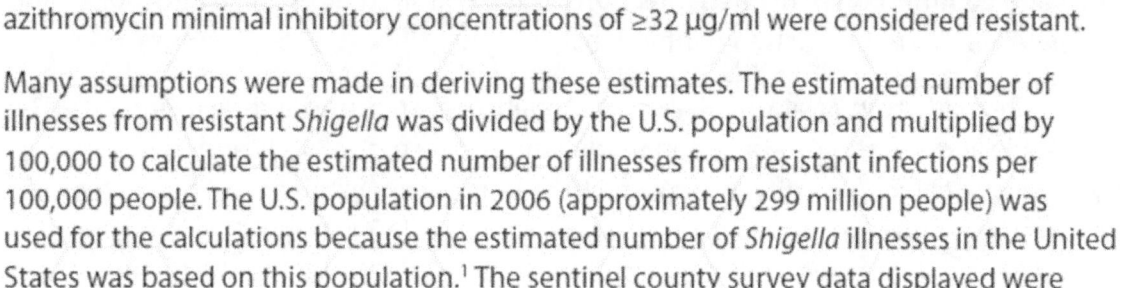

Methods

Estimates of the number of illnesses and deaths from infections with *Shigella* resistant to azithromycin or ciprofloxacin are reported. They were derived by multiplying an estimate of the annual number of *Shigella* illnesses or deaths in the United States[1] by the prevalence of resistance among *Shigella* tested by the National Antimicrobial Resistance Monitoring System (NARMS) in 2011, the year azithromycin testing began. Resistance breakpoints from the NARMS 2011 Human Isolates Report were used.[2] As clinical azithromycin breakpoints have not been established for *Shigella*, the values used here were based on epidemiological cut-off values used in the NARMS report. Isolates with azithromycin minimal inhibitory concentrations of ≥32 µg/ml were considered resistant.

Many assumptions were made in deriving these estimates. The estimated number of illnesses from resistant *Shigella* was divided by the U.S. population and multiplied by 100,000 to calculate the estimated number of illnesses from resistant infections per 100,000 people. The U.S. population in 2006 (approximately 299 million people) was used for the calculations because the estimated number of *Shigella* illnesses in the United States was based on this population.[1] The sentinel county survey data displayed were previously reported.[3,4,5]

References

1   Scallan E, Hoekstra RM, Angulo FJ, et al. Foodborne illness acquired in the United States—major pathogens. Emerg Infect Dis 2011;17:7–15.

2   CDC. National Antimicrobial Resistance Monitoring System for Enteric Bacteria (NARMS): Human Isolates Final Report, 2011. Atlanta, Georgia: U.S. Department of Health and Human Services, CDC, 2013.

3   Tauxe RV, Puhr ND, Wells JG, Hargrett-Bean N, Blake PA. Antimicrobial resistance of *Shigella* isolates in the USA: the importance of international travelers. J Infect Dis 1990;162:1107–11.

4   CDC. National Antimicrobial Resistance Monitoring System for Enteric Bacteria (NARMS): 2003 Human Isolates Final Report. Atlanta, Georgia: U.S. Department of Health and Human Services, CDC, 2006.

5   Sivapalasingam S, Nelson JM, Joyce K, et al. High prevalence of antimicrobial resistance among *Shigella* isolates in the United States tested by the National Antimicrobial Resistance Monitoring System from 1999 to 2002. Antimicrob Agents Chemother 2006;50:49–54.

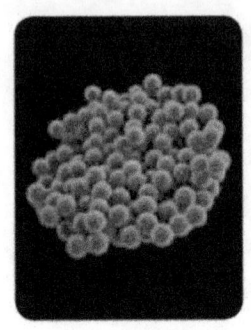

Technical Appendix

Methicillin-Resistant *Staphylococcus aureus* (MRSA)

Methods

National estimates of the number of invasive MRSA healthcare-associated infections (HAIs) were derived from the Emerging Infection Program/Active Bacterial Core Surveillance[1] for Invasive MRSA using data reported for infections occurring during 2011 (http://www.cdc.gov/abcs/reports-findings/surv-reports.html). During 2011, 4,872 reports of invasive MRSA (isolates of MRSA cultured from a normally sterile site and identified by a participating clinical laboratory) were received from the 9 participating program sites (population of 19,393,677). Reports include both healthcare-associated infections and community-associated infections, but are limited to invasive infections (approximately 85% are bloodstream infections).

Estimates were made using National Center for Health Statistics bridged-race vintage 2011 post-censal file and U.S. renal data systems, adjusting for race, age, gender, and receipt of dialysis. Mortality includes all-cause mortality during hospitalization, and estimates were adjusted in similar fashion as infection estimates. Approximately 18% of cases were reported without a race value, multiple imputation was used to estimate the missing race based on the data that are available and the results were summarized. Regarding device and procedure-associated infections with MRSA, the proportion of facilities reporting at least one *S. aureus* HAI reported as MRSA for each HAI type was obtained from CDC's National Healthcare Safety Network Antimicrobial Resistance Report 2009–2010.[2] Estimates were rounded to two significant digits.

References

1   Kallen AJ, Mu Y, Bulens S, Reingold A, Petit S, Gershman K, Ray SM, Harrison LH, Lynfield R, Dumyati G, Townes JM, Schaffner W, Patel PR, Fridkin SK; Active Bacterial Core surveillance (ABCs) MRSA Investigators of the Emerging Infections Program. Health care-associated invasive MRSA infections, 2005–2008. JAMA. 2010

2   Sievert DM, Ricks P, Edwards JR, Schneider A, Patel J, Srinivasan A, Kallen A, Limbago B, Fridkin S; National Healthcare Safety Network (NHSN) Team and Participating NHSN Facilities. Antimicrobial-resistant pathogens associated with healthcare-associated infections: summary of data reported to the National Healthcare Safety Network at the Centers for Disease Control and Prevention, 2009–2010. Infect Control Hosp Epidemiol. 2013 Jan;34(1):1–14

Vancomycin-Resistant *Staphylococcus aureus*

Methods

Vancomycin resistant *S. aureus* (VRSA) have been a nationally notifiable condition since 2004.[1] The national estimate of the number of VRSA cases is derived from individual case reports and confirmation at the Centers for Disease Control and Prevention (CDC). All reported VRSA are submitted to CDC for confirmatory antimicrobial susceptibility with reference broth microdilution.[2] Vancomycin resistance in *S. aureus* is defined as an MIC ≥ 16 ug/ ml. All isolates meeting this criterion are further characterized with PCR to detect known resistance mechanisms. All 13 U.S. VRSA identified to date have carried the *vanA* resistance determinant.[3]

References

1   http://wwwn.cdc.gov/nndss/document/nndss_event_code_list_2013.pdf

2   CSLI. 2012. Performance Standards for Antimicrobial Susceptibility Testing; Twenty-second Informational Supplement. Clinical and Laboratory Standards Institute, Wayne, PA

3   http://www.cdc.gov/HAI/settings/lab/vrsa_lab_search_containment.html

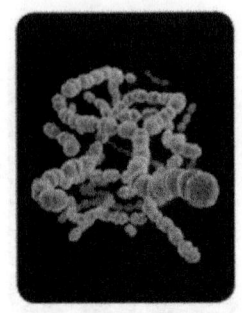

Methods

Trends in the incidence of antibiotic-resistant invasive pneumococcal disease per 100,000 persons are from Active Bacterial Core surveillance (ABCs), which is part of CDC's Emerging Infections Program (EIP) network.[1] ABCs conducts surveillance for invasive bacterial infections, including *Streptococcus pneumoniae*, at 10 sites located throughout the United States representing a population of approximately 30 million persons. Isolates are collected on ≥90% of all cases (approximately 3200 isolates per year) and sent to reference laboratories for susceptibility testing to eighteen different antibiotics using Clinical and Laboratory Standards Institute (CLSI) methods. Estimates of invasive pneumococcal disease are also from ABCs.[2]

Estimates of the burden of antibiotic resistant pneumococcal disease are derived from three sources. First, numbers of cases were estimated by applying the rate for full resistance to clinically relevant drugs (i.e. penicillin, ceftriaxone, cefotaxime, erythromycin, levofloxacin, tetracycline, trimethoprim/sulfamethoxazole) in 2011 (30%) to estimates of cases of all *S. pneumoniae* infections (4 million) as estimated by Huang and colleagues.[3] Numbers of deaths were estimated by applying the rate of full resistance to a clinically relevant drug (33%) to the total number of deaths from pneumococcal disease.[3] Excess pneumococcal pneumonia visits, hospitalizations, and costs were estimated using the previous overall burden estimates[3] but consideration of the burden of disease that would have occurred in the absence of resistance to penicillin, erythromycin, and levofloxacin.[4]

References

1   CDC. Active Bacterial Core Surveillance Methodology (2012). http://www.cdc.gov/abcs/index.html [Accessed 5/23/2013].

2   CDC. Active Bacterial Core Surveillance (ABCs) Report, Emerging Infections Program network, *Streptococcus pneumoniae* (2011). http://www.cdc.gov/abcs/reports-findings/survreports/spneu11.pdf [Accessed 5/23/2013].

3   Huang SS, Johnson KM, Ray GT, et al. Healthcare utilization and cost of pneumococcal disease in the United States. Vaccine 2011;29(18):3398-412.

4   Murphy CR, Finkelstein JA, Ray GT, Moore MR, Huang SS. Attributable Healthcare Utilization and Cost of Pneumonia due to Drug-Resistant *Streptococcus pneumoniae*. In: IDWeek; 2012 October 19, 2012; San Diego, CA: Infectious Diseases Society of America; 2012.

Technical Appendix

Erythromycin-Resistant Group A *Streptococcus*

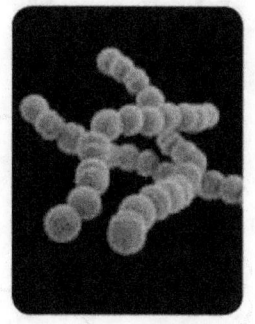

Methods

Estimates of the proportion of GAS isolates resistant to erythromycin, clindamycin and tetracycline are from isolates collected through Active Bacterial Core surveillance (ABCs), which is part of CDC's Emerging Infections Program (EIP) network.[1] ABCs conducts surveillance for invasive bacterial infections, including GAS, at 10 sites located throughout the United States representing a population of approximately 32 million people. Isolates are collected on ~80% of all cases (approximately ~1000 isolates per year) and sent to reference laboratories for susceptibility testing to twelve different antibiotics using Clinical and Laboratory Standards Institute (CLSI) methods.

Cases and deaths were estimated by applying 2011 resistant rate to erythromycin (10%, see Strep Group A *Streptococcus* pathogen page) to total cases (13300) and total deaths (1,550) reported in the 2011 report of the Active Bacteria Core surveillance (ABCs).[2]

References

1   CDC, Active Bacterial Core Surveillance Methodology (2012). http://www.cdc.gov/abcs/index.html [Accessed 5/23/2013].

2   http://www.cdc.gov/abcs/reports-findings/survreports/gas11.html

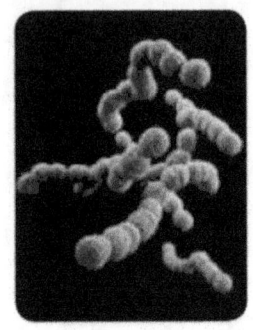

Methods

Estimates of the proportion of GBS isolates resistant to erythromycin and clindamycin are from isolates collected through Active Bacterial Core surveillance (ABCs), which is part of CDC's Emerging Infections Program (EIP) network.[1] ABCs conducts surveillance for invasive bacterial infections, including GBS, at 10 sites located throughout the United States representing a population of approximately 32 million persons. Isolates are collected currently from 7 of these states, from ~85% of the cases in these states (approximately ~1500 isolates per year) and sent to reference laboratories for susceptibility testing to twelve different antibiotics using Clinical and Laboratory Standards Institute (CLSI) methods. Estimates of severe disease are also from ABCs.[2]

Cases and deaths were estimated by applying the 2010 overall resistant rate to clindamycin (28%) from the ABCs antimicrobial susceptibilities report[3] to total cases (27,000) and total deaths (1,575) reported in the 2011 ABCs GBS surveillance report.[2]

References

1   CDC. Active Bacterial Core Surveillance Methodology (2012). http://www.cdc.gov/abcs/index.html [Accessed 5/23/2013].

2   CDC. Active Bacterial Core Surveillance (ABCs) Report, Emerging Infections Program network, Group B *Streptococcus* (2011). http://www.cdc.gov/abcs/reports-findings/survreports/gbs11.pdf [Accessed 7/23/2013].

3   CDC. Antimicrobial Susceptibilities Among Group B *Streptococcus* Isolates, Active Bacterial Core Surveillance (ABCs) (2010). http://www.cdc.gov/abcs/reports-findings/survreports/gbs10-suscept.html [Accessed 7/23/2013].

Glossary

All glossary definitions are from the CDC (2013) unless indicated otherwise by a citation at the end of the definition.

Active Bacterial Core surveillance (ABCs): A core component of CDC's Emerging Infections Programs network (EIP), a collaboration between CDC, state health departments, and universities. ABCs is an active laboratory- and population-based surveillance system that tracks invasive bacterial pathogens of public health importance. It currently operates among 10 EIP sites across the United States, representing a population of approximately 41 million persons. At this time, ABCs conducts surveillance for six pathogens: group A and group B *Streptococcus* (GAS, GBS), *Haemophilus influenzae, Neisseria meningitidis, Streptococcus pneumoniae,* and methicillin-resistant *Staphylococcus aureus* (MRSA).

Adverse drug event: When therapeutic drugs (example, antibiotics) have harmful effects; when someone has been harmed by a medication.

Aminoglycoside: A type of antibiotic that destroys the functioning of gram-negative bacteria. Increased resistance to aminoglycosides has made them less useful.

Antibiotic: Type of medicine made from mold or bacteria that kills or slows the growth of other bacteria. Examples include penicillin and streptomycin. (CDC 2013)

"How did and how do all these drugs perform their miracles? Antibiotics work in three general ways. One, as exemplified by penicillin and its descendants, is by attacking the machinery used by bacteria to create their cell walls…The second mechanism is inhibiting the way bacteria make the proteins that perform all of the important functions of the bacterial cell. The third is interfering specifically with the ability of bacteria to divide and reproduce, thereby inhibiting their doubling. With slower growth, they become less of a threat so the host can mount an immune response to deal with them more easily…A one-week course of an antibiotic can lead to persistence of resistant organisms more than three years later and in sites far away from the intended target of the antibiotic." (Blaser 2015)

Antibiotic class: A grouping of antibiotics that are similar in how they work and how they are made.

Antibiotic growth promotion: Giving farm animals antibiotics to increase their size in order to produce and sell more meat.

Antibiotic resistance: The result of bacteria changing in ways that reduce or eliminate the effectiveness of antibiotics. Antibiotic resistance is one type of antimicrobial resistance. (CDC 2013)

Resistance "spreads within bacterial communities in two general ways. First, it occurs through the growth of organisms that have already acquired resistance—what we call vertical transmission…Resistant genes can also transfer via sex, what we call horizontal transmission. Some bacteria are reclusive and many bacterial species are promiscuous and having sex all the time." (Blaser 2015)

Antibiotic stewardship: Coordinated efforts and programs to improve the use of antimicrobials. For example, facilities with antibiotic stewardship programs have made a commitment to always use antibiotics appropriately and safely—only when they are needed to prevent or treat disease, and to choose the right antibiotics and to administer them in the right way in every case.

Antimicrobial: A general term for the drugs, chemicals, or other substances that either kill or slow the growth of microorganisms. Among the antimicrobial agents in use today are antibacterial drugs (which kill bacteria), antiviral agents (which kill viruses), antifungal agents (which kill fungi), and antiparisitic drugs (which kill parasites).

Antimicrobial resistance: The result of microorganisms changing in ways that reduce or eliminate the effectiveness of drugs, chemicals, or other agents used to cure or prevent infections. In this report, the focus is on antibiotic resistance, which is one type of antimicrobial resistance.

Azithromycin: A macrolide antibiotic used to treat infections caused by gram-positive bacteria and infections such as respiratory tract and soft-tissue infections.

Azoles: A large class of drugs developed to treat fungal infections.

Bacteria: Single-celled organisms that live in and around us. Bacteria can be helpful, but in certain conditions can cause illnesses such as strep throat, ear infections, and bacterial pneumonia.

Bacteriology: The study of bacteria.

Beta (β)-lactamase enzyme: A chemical produced by certain bacteria that can destroy some kinds of antibiotics.

Biofilm: "There are microbes that can form gelatin-like layers surrounding themselves. These thick gels are called biofilms. Their composition varies, but biofilms can protect the barrier from drying out or from excessive heat, or from the onslaught of immunity." (Blaser 2015)

Broad-spectrum antibiotic: An antibiotic that is effective against a wide range of bacteria.

Carbapenem: A type of antibiotic that is resistant to the destructive beta-lactamase enzyme of many bacteria. Carbapenems are used as a last line of defense for many bacteria, but increased resistance to carbapenems has made them less useful.

Cefixime: A cephalosporin antibiotic that is resistant to the destructive beta-lactamase enzyme of many bacteria.

Ceftriaxone: A cephalosporin antibiotic that is resistant to the destructive beta-lactamase enzyme of many bacteria.

Celiac disease: An autoimmune disorder of the small intestine. "It is plausible that Celiac disease is increasing because the microbes that protect against allergic response are disappearing…People who had recently developed Celiac disease were 40% more likely to have been prescribed antibiotics in the preceding months." (Blaser 2015)

Cephalosporin: Cephalosporins are a class of antibiotics containing a large number of drugs. Some more recently developed cephalosporins are resistant to the destructive beta-lactamase enzyme produced by many bacteria.

Ciprofloxacin: A broad-spectrum fluoroquinolone antibiotic that is important in treating serious bacterial infections, especially when resistance to older antibiotic classes is suspected.

Clindamycin: An antibiotic used to treat certain types of bacterial infections, including infections of the lungs, skin, blood, female reproductive organs, and internal organs.

Conjugate vaccine: A vaccine in which an antigen is attached to a carrier protein from the same microorganism. This approach enhances the immunological response to the vaccine and thereby enhances the overall effectiveness of the vaccine.

Diabetes: A group of metabolic diseases that have high blood sugar levels. "The rate of type 1 diabetes is doubling every 20 years all over the developed world; moreover, children are coming down with the disease at younger ages…Kids with diabetes: lose weight rapidly, wet their beds, are constantly thirsty, and feel painfully exhausted." (Blaser 2015)

Echinocandins: A class of drugs developed to treat fungal infections.

EIP: The Emerging Infections Program network is a national resource for surveillance, prevention, and control of emerging infectious diseases. It was established in 1995.The EIP is a network of 10 state health departments and their collaborators in local health departments, academic institutions, other federal agencies, and public health and clinical laboratories; infection preventionists; and healthcare providers.

Emerging infections (EIs): Infections that have newly appeared in a population or have existed previously but are rapidly increasing in incidence or geographic range. (Morens 2004)

Endogenous flora: Bacteria that naturally reside in or on the body.

Epidemiology: The study of diseases to find out who is affected, how disease is spread, trends in illnesses and deaths, what behaviors or other risk factors might put a person at risk, and other information that can be used to develop prevention strategies. Epidemiologists use surveys and surveillance systems to track illnesses, and they often investigate disease outbreaks.

Erythromycin: An antibiotic used to treat certain infections caused by bacteria, such as bronchitis, diphtheria, Legionnaires' disease, pertussis (whooping cough), pneumonia, rheumatic fever, sexually transmitted diseases, and infections of the ear, intestine, lung, urinary tract, and skin. It is also used before some surgery or dental work to prevent infection.

Estrobolome: "The complete set of bacterial genes that code for enzymes capable of metabolizing estrogens within the human intestine." (themixuab.blogspot.com/2012/11/gut-bugs-relationship-with-estrogen.html)

Etiology of autism: "Multiple theories about to explain the increase in autism cases, including toxins in food, water and air; exposure to chemicals and pesticides during pregnancy; and particular characteristics of the fathers…My theory rests on the fact that gut microbes are involved in early brain development…Extensive studies point to abnormal serotonin levels in the blood of autistic children." (Blaser 2015)

Exotoxin: "A toxin secreted by bacteria. An exotoxin can cause damage to the host by destroying cells or disrupting normal cellular metabolism. Well-known exotoxins include botulinum [botulism], *diphtheriae* [diphtheria], and tetanospasmin [Clostridium]. The toxic properties of most exotoxins can be inactivated by heat or chemical treatment to produce a toxoid." (Wikipedia 2016)

Extended-spectrum antibiotic: An antibiotic that has been chemically modified to attack additional types of bacteria, usually those that are gram-negative.

Extensively drug-resistant (XDR): Resistance to nearly all drugs that would be considered for treatment. Exact definitions for XDR differ for each type of bacteria.

Fluconazole: An antifungal drug in the azole class.

Fluoroquinolones: Broad-spectrum antibiotics that play an important role in treatment of serious bacterial infections, especially hospital-acquired infections and others in which resistance to older antibacterial classes is suspected. Increasing resistant to fluoroquinolones is making them less effective.

Fungus: A single-celled or multicellular organism.Fungi can be opportunistic pathogens (such as aspergillosis, candidiasis, and cryptococcosis) that cause infections in people with compromised immune systems, such as cancer patients, transplant recipients, and people with HIV/AIDS.Fungi can also be or pathogens (such as the endemic mycoses, histoplasmosis and coccidioidomycosis, and superficial mycoses) that cause infections in healthy people. Fungi are used to develop antibiotics, antitoxins, and other drugs used to treat various diseases.

GISP: The Gonococcal Isolate Surveillance Project was established in 1986 to monitor U.S. trends in antimicrobial susceptibilities of strains of *Neisseria gonorrhoeae,* the type of bacteria that causes gonorrhea. The goal of GISP is to establish a rational basis for the selection of drugs used to treat gonorrhea. GISP is a collaborative project between selected sexually transmitted disease clinics, five regional laboratories, and CDC.

H. pylori: A bacterium found usually in the stomach. "As *H. pylori* is disappearing, stomach cancer is falling, but esophageal carcinoma is rising. It is a classic case of amphibiosi…*H. pylori*-induced immune cell populations protect against asthma…Could subclinical unrecognized cases of GERD caused by the lack of *H. pylori* be driving the asthma epidemic?" (Blaser 2015)

HAIs: Healthcare-associated infections are those that occur in hospitals, outpatient clinics, nursing homes, and other facilities where people receive care.

Hand hygiene: The practice of cleaning hands. This practice protects against infection and illness.

Hypervirulent: Increased ability to cause severe disease, relapse rates, and death.

Invasive disease: A disease that can spread within the body to healthy tissue.

Isolate/bacterial isolate: A pure culture or sample of bacteria used to study their properties.

Isoniazid (INH): A first-line drug used to treat tuberculosis. Strains of tuberculosis resistant to INH and rifampin are considered to be multidrug resistant.

Lactobacillus: A bacteria that makes the vaginal canal more acidic. (Wikipedia 2016)

Macrolide: A type of antibiotic used to treat infections caused by gram-positive bacteria and infections such as respiratory tract and soft-tissue infections. Macrolides are often used in people allergic to penicillin, but resistance to macrolides is increasing and has made them less useful.

Methicillin: An antibiotic derived from penicillin. It was previously used to treat bacteria such as *Staphylococcus aureus.*

Microbe: "Any living organism that spends its life at a size too tiny to be seen with the naked eye." (http://commtechlab.msu.edu/sites/dlc-me/zoo/ziwim.html)

Microbiology: The study of microorganisms.

Microorganism: Organisms so small that a microscope is required to see them. This term includes bacteria, fungi, parasites, and viruses.

Morbidity: The number of people who are infected with a specified illness in a given time period.

Mortality: The number of people who die in a given time from a specified illness.

MRSA: Methicillin-resistant *Staphylococcus aureus* is used to describe any strain of *S. aureus* that is resistant to all types of penicillin (not just methicillin) as well as cephalosporin.

Multidrug-resistant (MDR): Microorganisms that are resistant to multiple classes of antimicrobials. The exact number of drugs that a microorganism is resistant to varies depending on the infection or pathogen.

NARMS: The National Antimicrobial Resistance Monitoring System monitors antimicrobial resistance in foodborne and other enteric bacteria, including *Salmonella, Campylobacter, Shigella, Escherichia coli* O157, and *Vibrio* (non-*V. cholerae*). NARMS is a collaboration among CDC, the U.S.Food and Drug Administration (FDA), the U.S. Department of Agriculture (USDA), and state and local health departments.

Narrow-spectrum antibiotic: An antibiotic that is active against a limited range of bacteria.

NHSN: CDC's National Healthcare Safety Network is the nation's most widely used healthcare-associated infection tracking system. NHSN provides facilities, states, regions, and the nation with data needed to identify problem areas, measure progress of prevention efforts, and ultimately eliminate healthcare-associated infections. In addition, NHSN allows healthcare facilities to track blood safety errors and important healthcare process measures such as healthcare personnel influenza vaccine status and infection control adherence rates.

Outbreak: When a group of people develop the same illness around the same time, and the number of people affected is higher than normal. Outbreak investigations are conducted to identify what exposure the affected people had in common.

Pathogen: A microbe that makes you ill, popularly known as a "germ." (Wikipedia 2016)

Pan drug-resistance (PDR): Resistance to all drugs that would be considered for treatment.Exact definitions for PDR differ for each bacteria.

Penicillins: A class of antibiotics including amoxicillin, methicillin, piperacillin and other drugs based on the first true antibiotic discovered in 1928 by Dr. Alexander Fleming. Increased resistance has made many types of penicillins less useful.

Plastisphere: "A term used to refer to ecosystems that have evolved to live in human-made plastic environments." (Wikipedia 2016). "Recently, bacteria have been found munching on plastic particles floating in the open ocean. Although a slow process, at least 1,000 different species are involved in converting this 'plastisphere' to a healthier biosphere." (Blaser 2015)

Pneumonia: An inflammatory condition of the lungs affecting primarily the microscopic air sacs known as alveoli. It is usually caused by infection with viruses or bacteria, and typical symptoms include a cough, chest pain, fever, and difficulty breathing.

Prokaryote: A single celled organism that lacks a nucleus, e.g. bacteria. (Wikipedia 2016)

Reservoir: A person, animal, insect, plant, or other host that is carrying a pathogen (for example, bacteria or fungi) that causes infectious diseases. Some pathogens have animal reservoirs (to survive, they need animal hosts).Others pathogens have human reservoirs (to survive, they need human hosts).

Resistant bacteria: Microorganisms that have changed in ways that reduce or eliminate the effectiveness of drugs, chemicals, or other agents to cure or prevent infections.

Rifampin: A first-line drug used to treat tuberculosis. Strains of tuberculosis resistant to isoniazid (INH) and rifampin (RMP) are considered to be multidrug resistant.

Strain/bacterial strain: A strain is a genetic variant or subtype of a microorganism (for example, a flu strain is a subtype of the flu virus).Some strains of bacteria are resistant to antibiotics, and others are not. When bacteria become resistant to antibiotics, they can share their resistance with other bacteria to create new resistant bacterial strains.

Superinfection: An infection following a previous infection, especially when caused by microorganisms that are resistant or have become resistant to the antibiotics used earlier.

Surveillance: The ongoing systematic collection and analysis of data. Surveillance systems that monitor infectious diseases provide data that can be used to develop actions to prevent infectious diseases.

Susceptible bacteria: When antibiotics are effective at killing or stopping the growth of a certain bacteria, the bacteria is known as susceptible to antibiotics. Susceptible infections are infections that can be treated effectively with antibiotics.

Systemic agents: Drugs that travel through the bloodstream and reach cells throughout the body.

Tetracyclines: A class of broad-spectrum antibiotics including tetracycline, doxycycline, minocycline, and other drugs. Increased resistance has made many types of tetracyclines less useful.

Triclosan: 2,4,4' –trichloro-2'-hydroxyphenly ether. It is an antibacterial and antifungal agent found in consumer products. (Wikipedia 2016)

Vaccine: A product that produces immunity in a person's body and therefore protects them from an infectious disease. Vaccines are administered through shots, by mouth, and by aerosol mist.

Vancomycin: A drug that is frequently used to treat methicillin-resistant *Staphylococcus aureus* infections and that is also effective against other bacteria.

Vector: "In epidemiology, a vector is any agent (person, animal, or microorganism) that carries and transmits an infectious pathogen into another living organism." (Wikipedia 2016)

Virus: A strand of DNA or RNA in a protein coat that must get inside a living cell to grow and reproduce. Viruses cause many types of illness. For example, varicella virus causes chickenpox, and the human immunodeficiency virus (HIV) causes acquired immune deficiency syndrome (AIDS). (CDC 2013)

"Viruses are much smaller and simpler [than bacteria]. They require a host. They can only live within a cell, be it from a human or other animal, plant, or bacterium." (Blaser 2015)

Zoonotic disease (Zoonoses): Diseases transmissible from animals to humans. (Wikipedia 2016)

ACKNOWLEDGEMENTS

Many people in the CDC Office of Infectious Diseases (OID) contributed to this report. Their efforts are acknowledged below in alphabetical order.

National Center for Emerging Zoonotic and Infectious Diseases (NCEZID)

Beth Bell

Michael Bell

Anna Bowen

Chris Braden

Mary Brandt

Allison Brown

Ann Burkhardt

Denise Cardo

Tom Chiller

Angela Ahlquist Cleveland

Nicole Coffin

Michael Craig

Laura Eastham

Jason Folster

Scott Fridkin

Peter Gerner-Smidt

Patricia Griffin

Rosa Herrera

Martha Iwamoto

John Jernigan

Valerie Johnson

Marsha Jones

Cecilia Joshi

Maria Karlsson

Beth Karp

Fernanda Lessa

Shawn Lockhart

Shelley Magill

Cliff McDonald

Felicita Medalla

Martin Meltzer

Eduardo Mendez

Eric Mintz

Azizeh Nuriddin

John O'Connor

Benjamin Park

Jean Patel

Dana Pitts

Jared Reynolds

Scott Santibanez

Doug Scott

Elizabeth Skillen

Steve Solomon

Arjun Srinivasan

Robert Tauxe

Abbigail Tumpey

Michael Washington

Jean Whichard

Rachel Wolf

National Center for HIV/AIDS, Viral Hepatitis, STD, and TB Prevention (NCHHSTP)

Gail Bolan

Peter Cegielski

Harrell Chesson

Ann Cronin

Thomas Gift

Robert Kirkcaldy

Michael Iademarco

Suzanne Marks

Roque Miramontes

Rachel Powell

Robert Pratt

Maria Fraire Sessions

Wanda Walton

Hillard Weinstock

Jonathan Wortham

National Center for Immunization and Respiratory Diseases (NCIRD)

Ryan Gierke

Steve Hadler

Rana Hajjeh

Lauri Hicks

Lindsay Kim

Gayle Langley

Matt Moore

Alison Patti

Stephanie Schrag

Chris Van Beneden

Emily Weston

Cynthia Whitney

Jonathan Wortham

Appendix 2: Testimony to the Committee on Energy and Commerce, Subcommittee on Health, United States House of Representatives on Antibiotic Resistance and the Threat to Public Health by Thomas Frieden, Director of the Centers for Disease Control and Prevention

Good morning, Chairman Pallone and other distinguished members of the subcommittee. I am Dr. Thomas Frieden, Director of the Centers for Disease Control and Prevention (CDC), an agency of the Department of Health and Human Services, and I appreciate the opportunity to talk to you today about the public health threat of antibiotic resistance and the important role CDC plays in detecting, responding to and preventing this problem.

Introduction

Antimicrobials[1] are used to treat infections by different disease-causing microorganisms, including bacteria, mycobacteria, viruses, parasites and fungi. In the vast majority of cases where antimicrobials are used, the microorganisms have found a way to evade or resist the antimicrobial agent. Resistance occurs wherever antimicrobials are used -- in the community, on the farm, and in healthcare. Antimicrobial resistance is a global problem, and some of our most significant global threats are multi-drug resistant tuberculosis and drug-resistant malaria. Today, however, I will focus on domestic issues and antibiotic-resistant bacteria.

Antibiotic resistance is a public health problem of increasing magnitude, and finding effective solutions to address this problem is a critical focus of CDC activities. Infections with resistant bacteria were first reported over 60 years ago[2], but early on the problem was often overlooked, because if one antibiotic did not treat the infection another was usually available. Since then, infections with resistant bacteria have become more common in healthcare and community settings, and many bacteria have become resistant to more than one type or class of antibiotics. Consequently, doctors and nurses today are faced with treating infections where antibiotic options are very limited, and in some cases, where no effective antibiotics exist. When treatment options

are limited, healthcare providers might need to use antibiotics that are more expensive or more toxic to the patient. When no antibiotic is effective, healthcare providers may be limited to providing supportive care rather than directly treating an infection -- similar to how medicine was practiced before antibiotics were discovered. As resistance increases, the patient's risk of dying from infection also increases. Moreover, resistance is not just a problem for the patient who is infected. When an infection is not effectively treated because of resistance, the microorganisms will persist and potentially spread to others, further extending the resistance problem.

Antibiotics kill or inhibit bacteria that are susceptible to that antibiotic. Bacteria that are intrinsically resistant or that can acquire resistance will survive and replace the drug-susceptible bacteria. Thus, any antibiotic use will provide a selective pressure[3] that perpetuates resistant bacteria. The more that antibiotics are used, the greater the selective pressure. Antibiotics are the most important tool we have to control many life-threatening bacterial diseases once infection has occurred, yet increasing levels of resistance are compromising the effectiveness of these antibiotics. Bacteria have developed multiple ways of becoming resistant to antibiotics; the more often bacteria are exposed to antibiotics, the more likely they are to survive through one of these mechanisms. Antibiotics are used widely to treat persons in the community and in healthcare settings, and are also used to treat animals in agricultural settings. It is imperative that we assess the use of antibiotics carefully – regardless of setting -- and use them only when necessary, to avoid promoting the development of resistance among bacteria.

Antibiotic resistance is also an economic burden on the healthcare system. Resistant infections not only cost more to treat, but also can prolong healthcare use. In a 2008 study of attributable medical costs for antibiotic resistant infections, it was estimated that infections in 188 patients from a single healthcare institution cost between $13.35 and $18.75 million dollars.[4] Unfortunately, infections caused by antibiotic resistant bacteria are an everyday occurrence in healthcare settings.

Overview of CDC's Antibiotic Resistance Programs

Without continuing to improve on our response to the public health problem of antibiotic resistance, we are potentially headed for a post-antibiotic world in which we will have few or no clinical interventions for some infections. Addressing antibiotic resistance requires a multifaceted approach to reduce inappropriate use, prevent disease transmission, and develop new antibiotic agents. CDC's activities in this area are focused on two goals: preventing the emergence and spread of resistant organisms, and improving antibiotic use to reduce resistance. Many of these activities are conducted in collaboration with partners including other federal agencies, state and local public health departments, academic centers, and international organizations.

Disease Surveillance and Response

Disease surveillance is a core CDC activity. CDC uses surveillance systems to assess and monitor the scope, magnitude and trends of the antibiotic resistance problem.

Surveillance data are used not only to monitor resistance rates but are also used to drive and direct prevention efforts, determine treatment recommendations, guide new drug development, and evaluate the effectiveness of prevention programs. Several different surveillance tools have been developed for bacterial resistance because surveillance strategies and objectives vary for different problems. One of CDC's most important surveillance platforms is the Emerging Infections Programs (EIPs), a network of 10 state health departments working with collaborators in laboratories, healthcare facilities, and academic institutions to conduct population-based surveillance. Through population-based surveillance, CDC is able to provide national estimates of disease burden and to track changes in disease burden over time. Through this network, CDC conducts surveillance for both resistant communityassociated and healthcare-associated bacterial infections. Incidentally, the EIP network has been invaluable in our response to H1N1 influenza.

Another component of CDC's antibiotic resistance surveillance system is the National Healthcare Safety Network (NHSN). This web-based surveillance tool for hospitals and state health departments monitors healthcare-associated infections (HAIs), such as those caused by methicillin-resistant Staphylococcus aureus (MRSA), Clostridium difficile, and multi-drug resistant gram-negative bacteria. Over 2,500 U.S. hospitals (approximately half) are currently enrolled in NHSN, and the President's budget request for FY 2011 seeks to expand that enrollment by another 2,500 hospitals. Data from this network are used to monitor HAI rates and the prevalence of resistance among the bacteria causing infection.

The CDC, the Food and Drug Administration (FDA), and the Department of Agriculture (USDA) also work in collaboration with participating state and local health departments to operate the National Antimicrobial Resistance Monitoring System (NARMS). NARMS is a lab-based surveillance system in all 50 states that detects resistance in enteric bacteria (microorganisms that inhabit the intestines) that are commonly transmitted from animals to humans through food, such as Salmonella, Campylobacter, and E. coli. NARMS monitors trends in the prevalence of resistance among bacteria isolated from humans, retail meats, and livestock.

Preventing resistant infections provides the greatest opportunity to limit resistance. Strategies to prevent and control resistant bacteria vary by the pathogen and the setting in which the infection is acquired. For some diseases, like Streptococcus pneumonia, there are vaccines to prevent infections. For others, CDC works collaboratively to develop infection control and treatment guidelines. Prevention of HAIs, such as MRSA, resistant gram-negative bacteria,[5] and C. difficile, can require different interventions than those infections that are community-associated, such as tuberculosis and pneumococcal pneumonia. In all cases, surveillance data are used to monitor the effectiveness of prevention efforts.

CDC works with state and local public health authorities to detect and respond to the emergence of new resistant bacteria. Part of these efforts includes providing reference laboratory services for state and local public health departments to confirm and characterize unusual antibiotic resistance. New resistance patterns often require the development of new laboratory tools for detection. CDC develops these new laboratory tools and then distributes them widely to monitor resistance at the local level.

CDC also provides epidemiologic assistance in outbreak responses. Outbreaks caused by resistant bacteria can occur in community settings where people are concentrated, such as athletic teams, childcare centers, and prisons, or in healthcare settings, including hospitals, long-term care facilities, and ambulatory care facilities. In all of our investigations, CDC works cooperatively with state and local health authorities to learn from each outbreak and use the lessons learned to develop best practice recommendations to prevent similar outbreaks from occurring in the future.

Healthcare Associated Multi-Drug Resistant Gram-Negative Bacterial Infections
The newest resistance challenge in the healthcare setting is multi-drug resistant gram-negative bacteria. Particularly concerning are the carbapenemase-producing bacteria, such as bacteria of the Klebsiella species, among others. Bacteria with the carbapenemase-resistance trait are resistant to a class of drugs that were considered the "last resort" for treating serious infections caused by these bacteria. The antibiotic resistant traits are often located on mobile genetic elements, called plasmids. That means that resistance can be readily transferred from one bacterium to another, facilitating the spread of resistance between bacteria.

Most recently, CDC has collaborated with state health departments in New York, Illinois, Florida, California, and Arizona to address outbreaks of carbapenemase-producing Klebsiella. In addition to these outbreaks, our reference lab has confirmed carbapenemase-producing Klebsiella for 32 other States. Preventing the spread of these resistant bacteria is difficult because patients may harbor the resistant bacteria in their intestinal tracts, but this goes unrecognized because it does not make the patients sick. This is called "asymptomatic colonization." Outbreak investigations, such as the one CDC helped with at an Illinois long-term care facility, found that up to 50 percent of a patient population can harbor the resistant bacteria while only a few patients may have an active infection. Patients with asymptomatic colonization can be infectious without being sick themselves. There is no efficient method to identify all potential types of colonization; furthermore, many of these organisms are part of normal human bacteria, and simply eradicating them could harm a patient.

CDC has responded to this new public health threat by working with laboratory standard-setting institutions to identify and recommend tests for the accurate detection of carbapenemase-mediated resistance. CDC has also worked with our Healthcare Infection Control Practices Advisory Committee (HICPAC) to recommend methods to identify patients colonized with the resistant bacteria so that infection control precautions can be implemented to prevent further spread.

Acinetobacter is another species of gram-negative bacteria that causes infections in hospitalized patients and often becomes resistant to many antibiotics. Infected patients are usually the individuals with the most comprised health, such as those receiving intensive care. *Acinetobacter* has also caused a large number of infections among U.S. service members injured in the Middle East. CDC investigations of *Acinetobacter* have led to some important discoveries. First, these resistant bacteria can spread rapidly within a healthcare institution and between healthcare institutions within a community. Second, contamination of the hospital environment is often a significant contributor to the spread of the resistant bacteria. In turn, these discoveries have led to the development of aggressive infection control strategies for *Acinetobacter*. Fortunately, consistent application of rigorous infection control precautions and environmental cleaning practices can prevent the transmission of *Acinetobacter*.

MRSA Infections

MRSA infections are transmitted primarily in the healthcare setting. These infections were first encountered in healthcare settings in the 1980s, and the rate of infections has continued to rise. Reducing MRSA infection rates in U.S. hospitals is the focus of several local, regional, and national interventions. For example, the Veterans Affairs Pittsburgh Healthcare System, in collaboration with CDC, achieved a 60 percent reduction in the rate of MRSA infections after it implemented a series of infection control procedures based on evidence-based guidelines designed to decrease the transmission of MRSA in hospitals. The measures included strict attention to hand hygiene, enhanced surveillance for infections, effective use of isolation rooms, and behavior modification techniques for healthcare workers to emphasize the importance of the new procedures. These interventions were subsequently implemented in Department of Veterans Affairs (VA) medical centers nationwide and in multiple other healthcare systems.

National data from the NHSN show that there has been a significant drop in the incidence of both MRSA and methicillin-susceptible S. aureus (MSSA) central line-associated bloodstream infections among intensive care unit patients in U.S. hospitals over the last five years. The incidence of MRSA bloodstream infections per 1,000 central line days (i.e. a measurement of infection burden derived from the number of patients who have a central line, or catheter, whether infected or not) decreased by 50 percent, while the incidence of central line-associated MSSA infections decreased even more substantially, by 70 percent. Serious MRSA infections are also monitored using the Active Bacterial Core Surveillance (ABCs) system; a surveillance system conducted in the EIP network. MRSA ABCs data for 2005-2008 also show a decrease in hospital-onset and healthcare-associated MRSA infections, confirming a downward trend. Thus, it appears that these practical efforts to reduce the transmission of MRSA in hospitals are working, thereby reducing the need for antibiotic usage.

Most serious MRSA infections, an estimated 85%, are associated with a healthcare exposure, but nearly 14% of the infections are community-associated. Although progress in controlling MRSA in hospitals is being made, CDC ABCs data indicate that community-associated MRSA infections are not decreasing. Most of these are skin infections, but severe and sometimes fatal cases of necrotizing pneumonia continue to be reported among otherwise healthy people in the community with no links to the healthcare system. Controlling MRSA in community settings is a new challenge, and CDC is continuing to evaluate evidence-based methods to reduce these infections in community settings. While progress continues to be made, more can be done, and CDC wants every healthcare institution to move toward elimination of MRSA and all other HAIs.

Clostridium difficile

C. difficile infections can be an adverse consequence of antibiotic use. *C. difficile* bacteria can live in the intestinal tract without causing disease because its numbers are kept low by competing with healthy intestinal bacteria for nutrients. However, antibiotics can disrupt this balance by killing off healthy intestinal bacteria, *whereas C. difficile*, which is intrinsically resistant to many commonly used antibiotics, flourish and multiply. *C. difficile* disease can range from mild diarrhea to lifethreatening infections. Since 2000, the United States has seen a rapid increase in the number and severity of *C. difficile* infections, primarily in hospitalized patients. Studies done in collaboration with CDC have demonstrated that modifying antibiotic usage in healthcare facilities can decrease *C. difficile* disease rates. Other studies have shown that daily cleaning of hospital rooms will also significantly decrease *C. difficile* infection rates.

Gonorrhea

Over time, Neisseria gonorrhoeae (gonorrhea) has become resistant to every antibiotic that has been used to treat it. During the 1970s and 1980s, resistance to penicillin and tetracycline increased significantly, leading CDC to stop recommending those antibiotics for therapy. Over the past decade, fluoroquinolone-resistant gonorrhea spread from the Far East and Western Pacific to the United States, leaving only one class of antibiotics still recommended for effective gonorrhea treatment, the cephalosporins.

It is expected that gonorrhea will also acquire resistance to the cephalosporins. Strains with decreased susceptibilities to cephalosporins identified in laboratory testing and some treatment failures following therapy with oral cephalosporins have been reported from several countries in Asia. Cephalosporin resistance has not yet been reported in the United States and has not been detected by CDC. With over 330,000 cases reported each year in the US, even small changes in the treatment of gonorrhea (e.g., the need for multi-dose or multi-drug therapy) could significantly impact the cost and effectiveness of control efforts for this infection.

CDC is collaborating with the World Health Organization (WHO) to maintain and strengthen its regional gonococcal resistance surveillance programs and to strengthen the laboratory and epidemiological capacity of countries, particularly in the Far East and Western Pacific regions where resistance has emerged in the past.

Foodborne bacterial infections

Non-typhoid *Salmonella* causes approximately 1.4 million cases of disease in humans in the United States each year. Patients with complicated or severe infections are treated with fluoroquinolones or cephalosporins, and of these two drug classes, only cephalosporins are approved for treatment of children with these infections. Since NARMS began surveillance in 1996, cephalosporin resistance among *Salmonella* isolated from humans has increased significantly, and resistance to this class of drugs has also been found among *Salmonella* isolated from the livestock and retail meats for which NARMS conducts surveillance. In many cases, the same types of bacteria and genetic mechanisms of resistance are found in both human and animal sources. Studies have shown that use of cephalosporins in food animals can select for antibiotic resistant bacteria, and, in some cases, specific uses of this class of drugs in food animals are associated with higher rates of resistance among human Salmonella infections. In order to successfully manage resistance, it is important to understand antibiotic resistant human infections in the context of specific antibiotic use patterns, including use patterns in food animals.

Campylobacter is one of the leading causes of culture-confirmed foodborne bacterial disease in humans in the United States, and consumption of poultry has been shown to be an important risk factor for *Campylobacter* infection. Fluoroquinolones and macrolides are the drug classes of choice for treating *Campylobacter* infections. Following the approval of fluoroquinolones for use in poultry, rate of resistance to this class of drugs among human *Campylobacter* isolates rose sharply, to more than 20 percent. FDA has since withdrawn approval of this drug class for use in poultry, and NARMS continues to monitor *Campylobacter* from humans, retail meats and food

206

animals for fluoroquinolone resistance. Studies are also underway to understand domestic and foreign travel-associated sources of fluoroquinolone-resistant *Campylobacter*.

Tuberculosis

Treatment of drug-susceptible tuberculosis (TB) requires 6-9 months of therapy, while drug resistant cases require 18-24 months of therapy with drugs that are less effective, more toxic, and far more costly. TB bacilli become resistant to antibiotics through inappropriate or inconsistently taken therapy; therefore, programs that fail to assure appropriate prescription and direct observation of treatment regimens, drug susceptibility testing, uninterrupted drug supplies, and patient support throughout duration of therapy can contribute to the development of drug resistance. This was the scenario in the United States from 1985 to 1993. Due to a combination of program neglect, the HIV epidemic, and outbreaks in congregate settings, the United States experienced 52,100 more TB cases than otherwise would have been expected during this period. An influx of emergency funds enabled CDC to build capacity in state, local, and territorial health departments to implement Directly Observed Therapy, where healthcare or outreach workers observe the taking of each dose of anti-TB medication and monitor patients' response.

As a result, TB incidence in the United States has declined from 25,107 cases in 1993 to a preliminary count of 11,540 in 2009, with proportional decreases in drug-resistant TB cases. In 2008, 1.1 percent of U.S. TB cases were drug resistant as compared with rates exceeding 20 percent in other parts of the world. [6] However, the epidemiology of drug-resistant TB in the United States has changed, reflecting global patterns. In 1993, 26 percent of multi-drug resistant TB cases occurred in foreign-born persons, whereas in 2008 this was 78 percent. 7 CDC monitors for drug resistance in the United States and, globally, collaborates with the United States Agency for International Development and WHO to provide technical assistance to national TB programs to monitor and prevent drug resistance and implement infection control practices in congregate settings, for example, in waiting rooms in HIV antiretroviral therapy clinics. CDC is also conducting research to develop shorter, more effective regimens for treating TB, drug-resistant strains, and TB in HIV-coinfected persons and children.

Pneumococcal Infections

Vaccination is effective in preventing pneumococcal infections. Penicillin-resistant pneumococcal infections became common during the 1990s. In 2000, a new pneumococcal conjugate vaccine became available for children in the United States, and CDC began tracking the vaccine's impact on resistant pneumococcal infections with the ABCs project. Since the vaccine was introduced into the routine childhood immunization program in the United States, penicillin-resistant pneumococcal

207

infections have declined by 35 percent. Not only has the vaccine been shown to prevent antibioticresistant infections, it has been shown to reduce the need for prescribing antibiotics for children with pneumococcal infection in the first place. CDC data also show that adults are getting fewer resistant pneumococcal infections because the vaccine is preventing spread of pneumococci from infected children to adults. It is estimated that since 2001, 170,000 severe pneumococcal infections and 10,000 deaths have been prevented by vaccine use and that the vaccine is highly cost-effective, saving an estimated $310 million in direct medical costs each year.

Despite the success of this vaccine, CDC's surveillance has identified the emergence of infections caused by a new multidrug-resistant strain of pneumococcus called serotype 19A. In a sense, the vaccine has provided selective pressure benefiting strains not covered by the vaccine. In February of this year, a new version of the vaccine, which includes protection against strain 19A, was approved for use. CDC will continue to use its surveillance systems to evaluate the impact of this new version of the vaccine.

Improving Antibiotic Use

Antibiotic use often provides lifesaving therapy to those who have a serious bacterial infection. Antibiotic use also provides the selective pressure for new resistance to develop. In order to minimize the selective pressure of antibiotics, it is important to make sure that when antibiotics are used, they are used appropriately. CDC's educational campaign **Get Smart: Know When Antibiotics Work** teaches both the provider and the patient when antibiotics should be used.

The **Get Smart: Know When Antibiotics Work** program is a comprehensive and multi-faceted public health effort to help reduce the rise of antibiotic resistance. Partnerships with public and private health care providers, pharmacists, a variety of retail outlets, and the media result in broad distribution of the campaign's multi-cultural/multi-lingual health education materials for the public and health care providers. Through **Get Smart**, CDC develops clinical guidance and principles for appropriate antibiotic use to prevent and control antibiotic-resistant upper respiratory infections. **Get Smart** targets five respiratory conditions that account for most of office-based antibiotic prescribing, including: otitis media, sinusitis, pharyngitis, bronchitis, and the common cold. Data from the National Ambulatory Medical Care Survey confirm the campaign's impact on reducing antibiotic use for acute respiratory tract infections among both children and adults. There has been a 20 percent decrease in prescribing for upper respiratory infections (In 1997 the prescription rate for otitis media in children less than 5 years of age was 69 prescriptions per 100 children compared to 47.5 per 100 children in 2007.) and a 13 percent decrease in prescribing overall for all office visits (Overall antibiotic prescribing dropped from 13.8

prescriptions per 100 office visits to 12.0 prescriptions per 100 office visits, comparing 1997-98 to 2005-06) 8 . The **Get Smart: Know When Antibiotics Work** campaign contributed to surpassing the Healthy People 2010 target goal to reduce the number of antibiotics prescribed for ear infections in children under age 5.

Following the success of this campaign, two new **Get Smart** campaigns have been launched: **Get Smart in Healthcare Settings** and **Get Smart on the Farm**. **Get Smart in Healthcare Settings** will focus on improving antibiotic use for the in-patient population. One of the initial activities will be to launch a website that will provide healthcare providers with materials to design, implement, and evaluate antibiotic stewardship interventions locally. These materials will include best practices from established and successful hospital antibiotic stewardship programs.

Antibiotics are also used in veterinary medicine and animal agriculture. Antibiotic use in animals has lead to the emergence of resistant bacteria, and sometimes these resistant bacteria can be transferred from animals to humans by direct contact or by handling and/or consuming contaminated food. Get Smart: Know When Antibiotics Work on the Farm is an educational campaign with the purpose of promoting appropriate antibiotic use in veterinary medicine and animal agriculture. CDC funds and provides technical assistance for several state-based efforts to educate veterinarians and food producers, including those in the dairy and beef industries.

There are several CDC initiatives to improve surveillance of antibiotic use to measure how much and where antibiotics are used. One initiative is an enhancement of the NHSN to accept antibiotic use data from healthcare facilities through electronic medical records. This capability is expected to be available in the next year. The second is a point prevalence survey of antibiotic use in selected healthcare facilities from around the U.S. This survey will be conducted through our EIP network, and it is expected to give us a snapshot of antibiotic use in the U.S. Antibiotic use data from both initiatives will provide much-needed information for implementing more targeted strategies to improve antibiotic use nationwide.

Antibiotic Resistance Requires a Coordinated Response

Since the impact of resistance is extensive, the Interagency Task Force on Antimicrobial Resistance was created to plan and coordinate federal government activities. The Task Force is finalizing an update of "A Public Health Action Plan to Combat Antimicrobial Resistance", which was first released in 2001. The Action Plan will focus on:

• reducing inappropriate antimicrobial use;
• reducing the spread of antimicrobial resistant microorganisms in institutions,

communities, and agriculture
• encouraging the development of new anti-infective products, vaccines, and adjunct therapies; and
• supporting basic research on antimicrobial resistance.

The Task Force is co-chaired by CDC, FDA, and the National Institutes of Health and includes seven other federal agencies (Agency for Healthcare Research and Quality, Centers for Medicare and Medicaid Services, USDA, Department of Defense, VA, Environmental Protection Agency, and Healthcare Resources and Services Administration).

Conclusion

With the growing development of antibiotic resistance, it is imperative that we no longer take the availability of effective antibiotics for granted. As a nation, we must respond to this growing problem, and our response needs to be multifactorial and multidisciplinary. CDC will continue to develop improved diagnostics to detect resistance rapidly and accurately. With the increased investments under the President's budget, we will enhance our surveillance systems, such as NHSN, with electronic laboratory data and electronic medical records data, which will facilitate surveillance at the healthcare level and thereby increase surveillance capacity. It will also result in real-time reporting, which means that there will be greater opportunities for a rapid prevention and control response. Healthcare institutions need robust infection control programs and antibiotic stewardship programs to prevent transmission of resistant bacteria and to decrease the selective pressure for resistance. CDC will continue its support of new and effective vaccines, like the pneumococcal vaccine, to prevent infections caused by some of the most serious infections such as MRSA and C. difficile. By building on our current efforts, we can extend the life of current antibiotics and develop future antibiotic therapies to protect us from current and future disease threats.

1 Antimicrobial is a general term for the drugs, chemicals, or other substances that either kill or slow the growth of microbes. Among the antimicrobial agents in use today are antibiotic drugs (which kill bacteria), antiviral agents (which kill viruses), antifungal agents (which kill fungi), and antiparisitic drugs (which kill parasites). An antibiotic is a type of antimicrobial agent made from a mold or a bacterium that kills, or slows the growth of other microbes, specifically bacteria. Examples include penicillin and streptomycin.

2 Barber M. Staphylococcal infections due to penicillin-resistant strains. British Medical Journal. 1947.

3 Selective pressure means that use of antibiotics will kill susceptible bacteria, but also "enrich" resistant bacteria. Resistant bacteria are "enriched" by the lack of susceptible bacteria to compete with for space,

resources, hosts, etc. Thus, those resistant organisms can often thrive and multiple, passing on their resistant genes to the next generation

4 Roberts, RR, Hota B, Ahmad I, Scott RD II, Foster SD, Abbasi F, Schabowski S, Kampe LM, Ciavarella GG, Supino M, Naples J, Cordell R, Levy SB, Weinstein, RA. Hospital and societal costs of antimicrobial-resistant infections in a Chicago teaching hospital: implications for antibiotic stewardship. Clin. Infect. Dis. 2009; 49:1175-84.

5 There are several types of gram-negative bacteria that cause healthcare-associated infections. Some of the more common bacteria belong to the Enterobacteriaceae family, such as Klebsiella spp., and Escherichia coli. Other important bacteria are Acinetobacter spp. and Pseudomonas aeruginosa.

6 MMWR, March 19, 2020/59(10), 289-294 and Multidrug and extensively drug-resistant TB (M/XDR-TB): 2010 global report on surveillance and response.WHO/HTM/TB/2010.3

7 CDC. Reported Tuberculosis in the United States, 2008. (http://www.cdc.gov/tb)

8 Unpublished data from the National Ambulatory Medical Care Survey, National Center for Health Statistics, 2009; http://www.cdc.gov/nchs/ahcd.htm

Appendix 3: Get Smart: Know When Antibiotics Work

From: http://www.cdc.gov/getsmart/community/materials-references/research-articles.html

The Get Smart: Know When Antibiotics Work program has developed an abbreviated list of recommended readings on the topic of appropriate antibiotic prescribing and use, as well as antibiotic resistance. Publications related to outpatient stewardship and clinical practice guidelines are located elsewhere on this website.

Adverse Drug Events

- Bourgeois FT, Mandl KD, Valim C, Shannon MW. Pediatric adverse drug events in the outpatient setting: An 11-year national analysis. *Pediatrics*. 2009; 124(4): e744–50.
- Budnitz DS, Pollock DA, Weidenbach KN, et al. National surveillance of emergency department visits for outpatient adverse drug events. *JAMA*. 2006;296(15):1858–66.
- Sarkar U, Lopez A, Maselli JH, Gonzales R. Adverse drug events in U.S. adult ambulatory medical care. *Health Serv Res*. 2011;46(5):1517–33.
- Schaefer MK, Shehab N, Cohen AL, Budnitz DS. Adverse events from cough and cold medications in children. *Pediatrics*. 2008;121(4):783–87.
- Shehab N, Patel PR, Srinivasan A, Budnitz DS. Emergency department visits for antibiotic-associated adverse events. *Clin Infect Dis*. 2008;47(6):735–43.

Antibiotic Resistance

- Antibiotic resistance threats in the United States, Centers for Disease Control and Prevention, accessed May 19, 2014.
- Antimicrobial resistance: Global report on surveillance 2014, World Health Organization, accessed May 19, 2014.
- Bronzwaer SL, Cars O, Buchholz U, et al. A European study on the relationships between antimicrobial use and antimicrobial resistance. *Emerg Infect Dis*. 2002;8(3):278–82.
- Earnshaw S, Mendez A, Monnet DL, et al. Global collaboration to encourage prudent antibiotic use. *Lancet Infect Dis*. 2013;13(12):100–34.

212

- Grijalva CG, Nuorti JP, Griffin MR. Antibiotic prescription rates for acute respiratory tract infections in US ambulatory settings. *JAMA*. 2009;302(7):758–66.
- Lipsitch M, Samore MH. Antimicrobial use and antimicrobial resistance: A population perspective. *Emerg Infect Dis*. 2002;8(4):347–54.

Antibiotic Resistance Efforts

- Hughes JM. Preserving the lifesaving power of antimicrobial agents. *JAMA*. 2011;305(10):1027–28.
- Huttner B, Goossens H, Verheij T, Harbarth S, on behalf of the CHAMP consortium. Characteristics and outcomes of public campaigns aimed at improving the use of antibiotics in outpatients in high-income countries[15 pages]. *Lancet Infect Dis*. 2010;10(1):17–31.
- A public health action plan to combat antimicrobial resistance: 2012 update[46 pages], Interagency Task Force on Antimicrobial Resistance, accessed May 19, 2014.
- Friedman CR, Whitney CG. It's time for a change in practice: Reducing antibiotic use can alter antibiotic resistance[2 pages]. *J Infect Dis*. 2008;197(8):1082–83.
- Strengthening U.S. antibiotic resistance efforts, Infectious Diseases Society of America, accessed May 19, 2014.

Knowledge, Attitude, and Practice Studies

- Barden LS, Dowell SF, Schwartz B, Lackey C. Current attitudes regarding use of antimicrobial agents: Results from physician's and parents' focus group discussions. *Clin Pediatr (Phila)*. 1998; 37(11):665–71.
- Butler CC, Rollnick S, Pill R, Maggs-Rapport F, Stott N. Understanding the culture of prescribing: Qualitative study of general practitioners' and patients' perceptions of antibiotics for sore throats. *BMJ*. 1998; 317(7159):637–42.
- Finkelstein JA, Dutta-Linn M, Meyer R, Goldman R. Childhood infections, antibiotics, and resistance: What are parents saying now? *Clin Pediatr (Phila)*. 2014;53(2):145–50.

- Mangione-Smith R, Elliott MN, Stivers T, et al. Racial/ethnic variation in parent expectations for antibiotics: Implications for public health campaign.*Pediatrics*. 2004;113(5):e385–94.
- Srinivasan A, Song X, Richards A, et al. A survey of knowledge, attitudes, and beliefs of house staff physicians from various specialties concerning antimicrobial use and resistance. *Arch Intern Med*. 2004;164(13):1451–56.
- Vanden Eng J, Marcus R, Hadler JL, et al. Consumer attitudes and use of antibiotics. *Emerg Infect Dis*. 2003;9(9):1128–35.

Prescribing Data

- Hicks L, Bartoces M, Roberts R, et al. US Outpatient Antibiotic Prescribing Variation According to Geography, Patient Population, and Provider Specialty in 2011. *Clin Infect Dis*. 2015;doi: 10.1093/cid/civ076.
- Barnett ML, Linder JA. Antibiotic prescribing for adults with acute bronchitis in the United States, 1996–2010. *JAMA*. 2014;311(19):2020–22.
- Centers for Disease Control and Prevention. Office-related antibiotic prescribing for persons aged ≤14 years — United States, 1993–1994 to 2007–2008. *MMWR*. 2011;60(34):1153–56.
- Fairlie T, Shapiro DJ, Hersh AL, Hicks LA. National trends in visit rates and antibiotic prescribing for adults with acute sinusitis. *Arch Intern Med*. 2012;172(19):1513-14.
- Grijalva CG, Nuorti JP, Griffin MR. Antibiotic prescription rates for acute respiratory tract infections in US ambulatory settings. *JAMA*. 2009;302(7):758–66.
- Hicks LA, Taylor TH, Hunkler RJ. U.S. outpatient antibiotic prescribing, 2010. *N Engl J Med*. 2013;368(15):1461–2.
- Linder JA, Bates DW, Lee GM, Finkelstein JA. Antibiotic treatment of children with sore throat. *JAMA*. 2005;294(18):2315–22.
- Mangione-Smith R, Wong L, Elliott MN, McDonald L, Roski J. Measuring the quality of antibiotic prescribing for upper respiratory infections and bronchitis in 5 US health plans. *Arch Pediatr Adolesc Med*. 2005;159(8):751–57.

- Shapiro DJ, Hicks LA, Pavia AT, Hersh AL. Antibiotic prescribing for adults in ambulatory care in the USA, 2007–09. *J Antimicrob Chemother*. 2014;69(1):234–40.

Appendix 4: Worldwide Tuberculosis Statistics

From: World Health Organization. (2016). *Tuberculosis*.
http://www.who.int/mediacentre/factsheets/fs104/en/

- Tuberculosis (TB) is a top infectious disease killer worldwide.
- In 2014, 9.6 million people fell ill with TB and 1.5 million died from the disease.
- Over 95% of TB deaths occur in low- and middle-income countries, and it is among the top 5 causes of death for women aged 15 to 44.
- In 2014, an estimated 1 million children became ill with TB and 140 000 children died of TB.
- TB is a leading killer of HIV-positive people: in 2015, 1 in 3HIV deaths was due to TB.
- Globally in 2014, an estimated 480 000 people developed multidrug-resistant TB (MDR-TB).
- The Millennium Development Goal target of halting and reversing the TB epidemic by 2015 has been met globally. TB incidence has fallen by an average of 1.5% per year since 2000 and is now 18% lower than the level of 2000.
- The TB death rate dropped 47% between 1990 and 2015.
- An estimated 43 million lives were saved through TB diagnosis and treatment between 2000 and 2014.
- Ending the TB epidemic by 2030 is among the health targets of the newly adopted Sustainable Development Goals.

Appendix 5: Commensals: Underappreciated Reservoirs of Antibiotic Resistance

Commensals: Underappreciated Reservoir of Antibiotic Resistance

Probing the role of commensals in propagating antibiotic resistance should help preserve the efficacy of these critical drugs

Bonnie M. Marshall, Dorothy J. Ochieng, and Stuart B. Levy

Antibiotic resistance, reported for sulfonamides in the mid-1930s and for penicillins in the 1940s, remains a stubborn quandary. What was once confined mainly to hospitals increasingly involves multidrug resistance that encompasses communities and encircles the globe. Virtually all types of bacterial infections are becoming resistant to antibiotic treatments, according to officials at the Centers for Disease Control and Prevention in Atlanta, Ga. Yet, despite decades of grappling with these issues, we still do not understand fully how genes carrying resistance traits spread, what makes certain species highly promiscuous in transferring those traits, whether there are effective barriers to their spread, and the frequency with which resistance genes move independently or in tandem with other migrating genes.

While evidence points to microorganisms associated with food, animals, and water as the main sources for resistance genes, which of them exerts the most impact is not known. We also do not know how important a role the burgeoning aquaculture industry plays, particularly in those countries where such farms are poorly regulated and may not only abuse antibiotics but sometimes even operate within the confines of wastewater treatment plants. Equally worrisome are the sludge products of urban and rural wastewater treatment plants that are increasingly used for fertilizer — dispersing unknown amounts of resistance genes and antibiotics that withstand standard sewage treatment.

In 2008, the Alliance for the Prudent Use of Antibiotics (APUA) convened microbiologists and other experts to review these and related questions and also to address the role of commensal and other nonpathogenic microorganisms in the overall problem of antibiotic resistance development and dis-

Summary

- Antibiotic resistance, increasingly dominated by multidrug-resistant microorganisms, is a growing threat to public health on a global basis.

- The Alliance for the Prudent Use of Antibiotics (APUA) is developing databases to track commensals and free-living microorganisms that provide a large reservoir for resistance genes that could transfer to pathogens (www.apua.org).

- A move to standardize methods and to improve surveillance systems, with emphasis on gene tracking, will help in analyzing antibiotic resistance.

- Multidisciplinary approaches, including gene-based technologies to study commensal ecology and a focus on aquaculture and wastewater environments, are needed to track resistance.

Bonnie M. Marshall is a Staff Scientist at The Alliance for the Prudent Use of Antibiotics and Research Associate in the Center for Adaptation Genetics and Drug Resistance and the Department of Molecular Biology and Microbiology, Tufts University School of Medicine, Boston, Mass. Dorothy J. Ochieng is a Project Manager at The Alliance for the Prudent Use of Antibiotics, and Stuart B. Levy is President of The Alliance for the Prudent Use of Antibiotics and Director of the Center for Adaptation Genetics and Drug Resistance and Distinguished Professor in the Departments of Molecular Biology and Microbiology and of Medicine, Tufts University School of Medicine.

persal. They concluded that a multidisciplinary ecological approach is imperative to tackling these resistance challenges (www.apua.org). Further, research and surveillance should not focus solely on strains and their phenotypic expression of resistance. They also urged investigators to use genetic fingerprinting to gain insights into sources of drug resistance genes and differences in strain behaviors under similar selective pressures. Probing commensals and understanding the role they play in antibiotic resistance should help toward developing effective interventions to control resistance and preserve the efficacy of antibiotics.

Blurred Border between Pathogens and Commensals

A classic example of expanding drug resistance comes from *Staphylococcus aureus,* which emerged with penicillin resistance soon after that drug was introduced. The pathogen later acquired resistance to methicillin and then to third-generation penicillins, and now additional antibiotics, including vancomycin, which is considered the drug treatment of last resort. Similarly, vancomycin-resistant strains of *Enterococcus faecium* are appearing globally. Like many other now-worrisome pathogens, these two bacterial species were once considered relatively harmless residents of the skin and intestinal tract that only sporadically caused problematic infections (Table 1).

Other multidrug-resistant bacteria are raising public health concerns. *Campylobacter* spp., which are indigenous to the intestinal tracts of many wild birds, and *Aeromonas* spp., which are native to aquatic environments, are infectious agents that increasingly bear multidrug resistance traits. Additionally, vancomycin resistance is appearing in microorganisms that, until recently, were rarely encountered as pathogens, including *Oerskovia turbata, Arcanobacterium haemolyticum, Streptococcus bovis, Streptococcus gallolyticus, Streptococcus lutetiensis, Bacillus circulans, Paenibacillus* spp., and *Rhodococcus* spp., as well as in the anaerobic genera *Clostridium* and *Eggerthella*. While not yet responsible for large-scale outbreaks, infections attributed to these species signify a worrying trend and pose the threat of disseminating resistance to vancomycin and other antimicrobial drugs to better-adapted pathogens.

People interact nonstop with microbes, most of them harmless or even beneficial. Some 26×10^{28} prokaryotes live in the top 8 m of soil, and another 12×10^{28} in aquatic environments, according to expert estimates. Additionally, 6 billion humans across the globe are colonized with an estimated total of 3.9×10^{23} microbes, of which pathogens constitute only a tiny fraction. Because commensals are widely viewed as harmless, support for their investigation has been scarce. The current Human Microbiome Project deviates sharply from that pattern.

Meanwhile, the heretofore disproportionate focus on antibiotic resistance in "true" and "opportunistic" pathogens was understandable —a consequence of the need to contend with the sequential appearance of resistance in microorganisms that cause illness. However, the associated monovision kept investigators from seriously examining other potential sources of resistance traits. Moreover, some of those other sources, such as anaerobic bacteria, were underappreciated and difficult to study. The blurring of their definition complicates the study of commensal flora. Escalating selective pressures, including those from antibiotic use and immunosuppressive therapies, further obscures boundaries, leading commensals into the realm of pathogens. This crossover phenomenon arises because the physical state of hosts has so much to do with defining which microorganisms are commensals and which are pathogens. A pathogen for one host can be a commensal for another host. Even so, defining a hierarchy for ranking commensals and pathogens helps in alleviating confusion and focusing research efforts (Fig 1).

Commensals Serve as Reservoirs of Resistance Genes

Commensals carry many types of resistance genes, which may be organized within genetic elements called integrons. Integrons carrying genes conferring resistance to older first- and second-generation antimicrobials are being recovered from nearly every type of environment. Moreover, integrons that carry resistance genes for the newer third- and fourth-generation antimicrobials are now appearing in diverse environments, including in commensal microorganisms associated with food animals and with humans (Table 2).

Finding resistance genes in microoganisms

within antibiotic-free environments suggests that those traits occur naturally and that they predate industrial-scale production and distribution of such drugs. Indeed, diverse and widely distributed soil bacteria carry resistance to virtually all antibiotics, including synthetic antimicrobials, some at clinically relevant concentrations, according to recent studies. These soil bacteria are phylogenetically disparate, and some of them are surprisingly close in genetic terms to human pathogens. Thus, on several grounds, these soil-dwelling microorganisms, with their reservoirs of antibiotic resistance traits, could be contributing to the rising levels of multidrug resistance now seen among pathogens that infect humans and other animals.

Escherichia coli and *Enterococcus* spp., which colonize humans and many other mammalian species, also are widely distributed throughout soil and water environments. Ubiquitous and resistant to a host of antibiotics, these species deserve serious attention. However, *E. coli*, which constitute only about 1% of the colonic flora, are outnumbered 20- to 30-fold by anaerobic *Bacteroides* spp. The remaining 70–80% of colonic flora consists of a staggering variety of species, mainly poorly characterized and comparatively ignored anaerobes that merit more scrutiny because they, too, can carry resistance genes. Meanwhile, other environments, particularly aquaculture, wastewater, and sludge, are mixing pots for the exchange of resistance traits and the emergence of novel strains carrying them (Fig. 2).

Our current multidrug resistance problem stems largely from horizontal gene transfers—a more efficient mechanism by which microorganisms adapt to environmental changes compared to random mutations. A growing body of evidence indicates that large quantities of genetic material, including antibiotic resistance genes, readily transfer among microbial species. Of the known gene transfer routes, transformation and conjugation appear to occur relatively frequently among densely packed cells of biofilms, such as those found in the intestinal tract and along tooth surfaces. In general, however, conjugation is perhaps the more common mechanism for lateral gene transfers. Little appears to inhibit this means of gene move-

Table 1. Emergence of antibiotic resistance in commensal bacteria causing disease[a]

Species	Disease	Year	Resistance
Acinetobacter baumanii	Nosocomial pneumonia, bacteremia, urinary tract infection, meningitis, septicemia	1985	Imipenem
		1993	Gentamicin
		1998	MDR[b]
		2001	Polymixin
Campylobacter jejuni	Campylobacteriosis	1986	Fluoroquinolone
Clostridium difficile	*Clostridium difficile*-associated diarrhea	1989	Clindamycin
Enterococcus faecalis	Endocarditis, bacteremia, catheter-related infection, intra-abdominal and pelvic infections.	1978	Gentamicin
		1986	Vancomycin
		1986	Gentamicin
		1986	Vancomycin
		1989	Ampicillin
		1989	Penicillin
		2000	Linezolid
Haemophilus influenzae	Bacteremic respiratory tract infections, meningitis, epiglottitis, osteoarthritis	1972	Ampicillin
		1975	Chloramphenicol/Tetracycline
		1975	Chloramphenicol
		1979	MDR
		1979	Chloramphenicol/Ampicillin
Klebsiella pneumoniae	Pyogenic liver abcess, bacteremia, RTI[c]	1983	Late Generation Cephalosporins
Pseudomonas aeruginosa	Opportunistic infections in immunocompromised patients	1985	Ceftazidime
		1987	Fluoroquinolone
		1988	Imipenem
Serratia marcescens	Nosocomial infections (UTI)[d]	1986	Fluoroquinolone
		1992	Carbapenem
Staphylococcus epidermidis	Infective endocarditis, IV catheter infections, bacteremia, CSF shunt infections, UTIs, osteomyelitis, vascular graft infections, prosthetic joint infections	1962	Methicillin
		1994	Rifamycin
S. haemolyticus	Septicemia, peritonitis, UTI, infective endocarditis	1984	Vancomycin
		1997	MDR
S. aureus	Boils, styes, furunculosis, pneumonia, mastitis, phlebitis, meningitis, urinary tract infections, osteomyelitis and endocarditis.	1942	Penicillin
		1960	Methicillin
		1976	MDR
		2000	Vancomycin
S. pneumoniae	*Streptococcus pneumoniae* infection	1967	Tetracycline
		1977	MDR
		1978	Macrolide

[a] Excerpted from K. E. Jones, N. G. Patel, M. A. Levy, A. Storeygard, D. Balk, and J. L. Gittleman, Nature **451**:990-994, 2008. Suppl. information at www.nature.com/nature.
[b] Ampicillin-chloramphenicol-trimethoprim/sulfamethoxazole.
[c] RTI, respiratory tract infections.
[d] UTI, urinary tract infections.

FIGURE 1

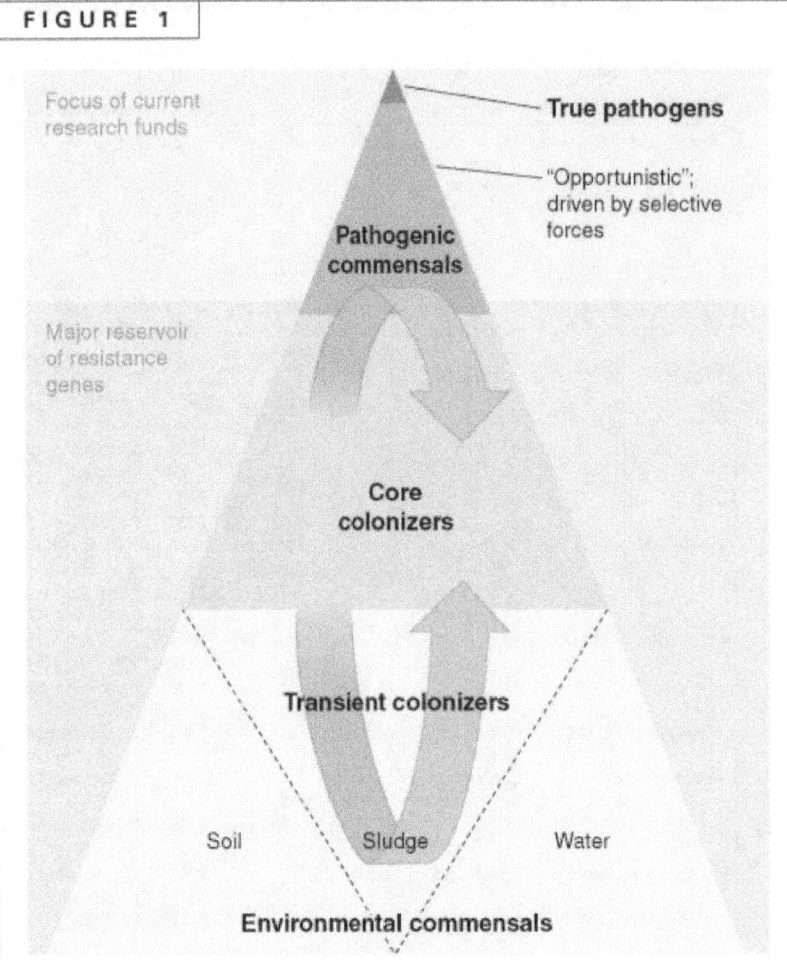

Focus of current research funds

True pathogens

"Opportunistic"; driven by selective forces

Pathogenic commensals

Major reservoir of resistance genes

Core colonizers

Transient colonizers

Soil   Sludge   Water

Environmental commensals

Hierarchy of commensals (not to scale). This group of microbes comprises only a tiny fraction of the total microbial environment. Greatly underated and understudied are the multitudes of "core" and transient colonizers, i.e., commensals that constitute the major reservoirs of resistance genes. To some degree, commensals can be distinguished by their place in the environment and the relationships with their hosts. Some colonizers of the skin, oropharynx, and intestinal tract rarely if ever cause disease (e.g., the lactic acid bacteria). Yet another group is considered generally nonpathogenic, but when imbalances or shifts occur in the selective pressures on their microbial niches, these species can be propelled to the status of pathogens, made more problematic if they have acquired resistance or virulence genes from neighboring commensals. These constitute the group of opportunistic or "pathogenic commensals." *Staphylococcus aureus*, which regularly or transiently colonizes about 80% of humans, now frequently crosses this border. *S. epidermidis* and other traditionally commensal coagulase-negative staphylococci only occasionally appear as nosocomial infections and only under extreme selective pressures, such as indwelling catheters and depressed immunologic states. Species that commonly harbor native or "constitutive" resistance in their chromosomes (e.g., *Pseudomonas*, *Stenotrophomonas*, and *Acinetobacter*), also may emerge under these conditions. Most commensals, however, exist as environmental residents of soil and water habitats, many of which may become transient colonizers of humans and animals through the food chain and other routes of exposure. The accumulated evidence suggests widespread gene exchange among these groups.

ment across dissimilar genera (Fig. 3). Transfer of antibiotic resistance genes from commensals to pathogens depends on the density of donor and recipient cells, the availability of a transfer mechanism, nutrition, and selective pressures. In this regard, the intestinal environment is considered optimal.

Gene cassettes within integrons, found in plasmids and chromosomes, are a major means for transporting and incorporating antibiotic resistance genes. Recently class 1 integrons, lacking antibiotic resistance genes, but bearing the phylogenetic signature of lateral gene transfer, were found on the chromosomes of nonpathogenic soil and freshwater *Betaproteobacteria*. Their close resemblance to class 1 integrons that are common among pathogens suggests that environmental *Betaproteobacteria* were an original source of these genetic elements.

ROAR Project Is Evaluating Commensals

While the medical community scrambles to handle emerging, drug-resistant superbugs, some investigators are pondering the origins of this resistance. The idea that resistance genes exist and appear clinically under selective pressures is a 30-year-old concept that was fueled by discovery of rare resistance genes within bacteria isolated from undisturbed environments. The gradual appearance of resistance in pathogens and subsequent demonstrations of widespread intergeneric gene migrations lent further credence to the idea that free-living microorganisms or commensal flora could be harboring transferable resistance genes. Another hypothesis is that genes converge, giving rise under special circumstances to de novo resistance genes.

During the 1990s, APUA began to examine commensals as possible carriers of antibiotic resistance genes through its Reservoirs of Antibiotic Resistance (ROAR) project, a collaborative effort that also involved Abigail Salyers of the University of Illinois in Champaign-Urbana. She and one of us (S.B.L.) along with other microbiologists suspected that commensal microorganisms were silently feeding drug resistance genes to species of clinical interest, making those commensals reservoirs of resistance genes.

To explore this possibility, ROAR began to focus on tracking the genes within commensal microorganisms, rather than the organisms themselves. If resistance was flowing from commensals to pathogens, tracking resistance genes could help to anticipate what might emerge among clinically important strains. The premise was that commensal flora could serve as barometers of resistance. However, the absence of global surveillance and standardized systems for phenotypic and genotypic tracking posed immediate challenges, which ROAR began to address by supporting research to fill some of these gaps. ROAR also began to support efforts to monitor resistance patterns in commensal bacteria (www.roarproject.org) and to envision other Web-based bioinformatics systems.

These efforts led directly to other challenges. For example, published information on commensals is scattered and difficult to track in part because microbiologists are not consistent in their use of the term. To remedy this problem, ROAR collected articles describing resistance in these populations, based on the following definition for commensals: "bacterial strains deemed not actively responsible for a pathogenic process and derived from humans, animals, or plants, or recovered from environmental sources such as air, water, soil, sludge, etc."

The ROAR collection of reports on commensals now includes more than 1,100 articles (published between 1969 and 2008), extracted from more than 260 journals. The reports describe isolates from 200 countries on all six continents that were collected between 1916 and 2008. They also describe more than 300 resistance genes and 144 virulence genes in species representing 66 different bacterial genera. The database is readily searchable and includes variables such as date, specific sources and sites where species were isolated, antibiotic exposure status, antibiotic susceptibility and multidrug resistance traits, and resistance transfer evaluations. Each annotation in the database can be linked directly to its PubMed citation.

Table 2. Detection of late-generation β-lactam resistance in commensal *E. coli* from different environments[a]

Resistance	Geographic site	Source	Frequency (%)
Bovines			
Amoxicillin-clavulanate	Canada	beef calves	3.9
		feedlot beef	1.2
	U.S. (Wisconsin)	Dairy cows	0.2/1.2[b]
Cefoxitin	Canada	beef calves	3.2
	U.S.	Dairy cows	0.7/0[b]
Ceftiofur	Canada	beef calves	2.9
		feedlot beef	0.7
	U.S.	Dairy cows	0.7/0[b]
	U.S. (Pennsylvania)	Dairy cows	11[c]
Cefoperazone	Great Britain	Abbatoirs	0.1
Swine			
Amox/clav	U.S. (8 states)	finishing farm	0.2/0.52[b]
	U.S. (Texas)	all/piglets only	2.2/6.8[b]
	Canada	Finishing farm	0.4–0.7
	Great Britain	Abbatoirs	0.2
	Thailand		5.8
Cefoxitin	U.S. (Texas)	all/piglets only	2.0/6.8[b]
	Canada	grow-finish farms	0.6–0.7
	Thailand		8.7
Ceftiofur	U.S. (8 states)	finishing farm	0.0/0.3[b]
	U.S. (Texas)	all/piglets only	2.4/7.1
	Canada	grow-finish farms	0.1
Ceftriaxone	U.S. (Texas)	all/piglets only	0.06/0.5
Ceftazidime	Great Britain	Abbatoirs	0.1
Cefoperazone	Great Britain	Abbatoirs	0.1
Sheep			
Amox/clav	Great Britain	Abbatoirs	0.2
Poultry			
Cefazolin	Korea		0.6
Cefoxitin	Korea		0.6
Humans			
Cefuroxime	Jordan		32
Cefazolin	Korea	Healthy students	0.6
Potable water			
Cefuroxime	Jordan		4

[a] Source: extracted from http://www.roarproject.org/
[b] Antibiotic-free/conventional.
[c] Ceftiofur used on 18% of farms surveyed.

Mining the ROAR Database

The ROAR review of commensal microorganisms is stimulating a wide range of questions regarding antibiotic resistance. However, the data needed to answer such questions are fragmentary at best. A key question is whether antibiotic use in agriculture and aquaculture is driving resistance genes from animal-associated bacteria into strains that cause human disease. Substantial but indirect evidence suggests that resistance genes pass from bacteria that colonize animals to bacteria associated with humans.

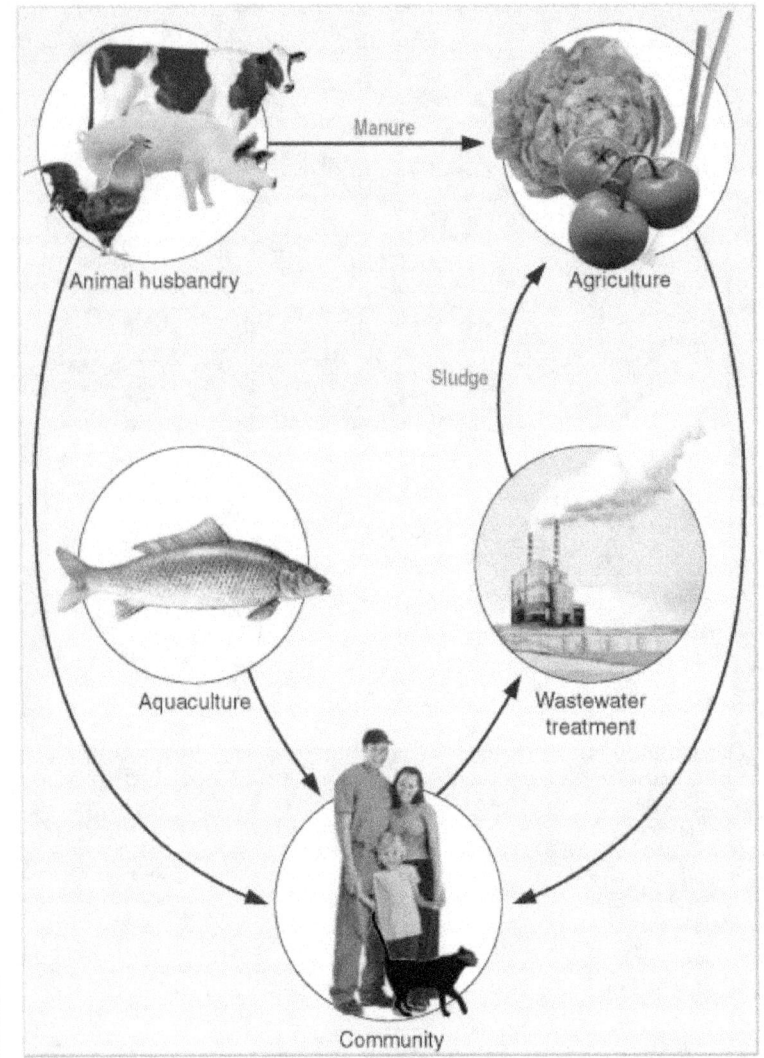

FIGURE 2

The interconnectedness of microbial communities and routes of transfer. Each arrow represents a route by which the simultaneous flow of commensals and pathogens can occur. Antibiotics are reported in varying concentrations in all these niches and act as selective agents on both pathogens and commensals. However, the complexities of these impacts have not yet been modelled. Note: In some countries, aquaculture occurs within the confines of sewage treatment facilities, creating a close link between these two environments.

to be so extensive, do not carry the same antibiotic resistance genes.

Strong evidence for direct transfers of antibiotic resistance traits from animal- to human-associated microorganisms comes from analysis of genera such as *Salmonella*, *Vibrio*, *Campylobacter*, *Yersinia*, and *Listeria*. They reside as commensals in many animal species, behaving as pathogens when humans consume raw, smoked, fermented, or undercooked foods. In such cases entire bacteria along with their resistance genes are transported from one host species to another. For example, when fluoroquinolones are used in poultry operations, humans exposed to those poultry food products pick up fluoroquinolone-resistant *C. jejuni* and become infected. However, there is still little direct evidence to show transfer of resistance genes from animal-associated *E. coli*, *Bacteroides*, or *Enterococcus* species into comparable human flora that subsequently cause antibiotic-resistant infections. The most persuasive evidence for this link remains a 20-year-old study in which the growth-promoting antibiotic nourseothricin (a streptothricin antimicrobial not used in human medicine) was used for two years as a feed additive for pigs on several neighboring farms. Plasmid-mediated streptothricin resistance was found in 33% of coliforms from pigs with diarrhea and also in 18% of pig farm employees and farm families, in 16% of healthy outpatients in that vicinity, and in 1% of urinary tract isolates from outpatients from surrounding communities.

Other studies support the idea that microorganisms associated with humans accumulate antibiotic-resistance genes from animal-associated microbes. For example, farmers and ranchers began using avoparcin, which is related to vancomycin, to supplement feed for livestock and poultry more than 20 years ago. Meanwhile, more and more vancomycin resistance has accumulated among enterococci, a commensal of the human gut, via Tn1546-like transfer elements. Slight differences in nucleotides

Similar resistance genes are being identified in dissimilar microbial species, implying that migrations and other changes occurred (Fig. 3). These migrations appear to be relatively recent because similar strains that were isolated earlier than 1970, which was before antibiotic use grew

from these mobile elements make it possible to determine whether the antibiotic-resistance genes in enteroccoci derive from commensals associated with swine or poultry. Again, the findings strongly implicate pork and poultry consumption as sources of these antibiotic resistance traits now common in human commensals.

Such evidence is not the same as direct tracking to prove the commensal connection. Direct approaches prove highly impractical, both ethically and because of requirements for long-term monitoring.

Predicting Emergence of Antibiotic-Resistant Pathogens

Antibiotic-resistance genes will transfer from commensals to pathogens in vitro with remarkable fluidity. For example, multiple resistance loci can transfer via conjugal means among commensal *E. coli,* pathogenic *E. coli,* and *Salmonella* strains in a simulated porcine ileum fermenter. However, predicting resistance trait transfers is difficult for many reasons, including vast differences in when they appear. For instance, resistance to penicillin appeared within a few years of its clinical use, whereas it took more than 30 years before vancomycin resistance began to appear in clinical isolates. These disparities undermine attempts to model antibiotic resistance on a general basis. Further, resistance is studied in depth in only a few microbial species, mainly *E. coli* and *Enterococcus,* adding to the difficulty in predicting how others might contribute, particularly anaerobic genera such as *Bacteroides* and *Clostridia.*

Meanwhile, it remains a formidable challenge to identify appropriate resistance genes to track in microorganisms in natural and agricultural settings and then to monitor for transfer into microbes associated with humans, including pathogens in clinical settings. In the absence of such direct experimental data, we plan to continue developing the ROAR database for monitoring commensal flora as an alternative means for analyzing how they contribute to the antibiotic resistance problem.

FIGURE 3

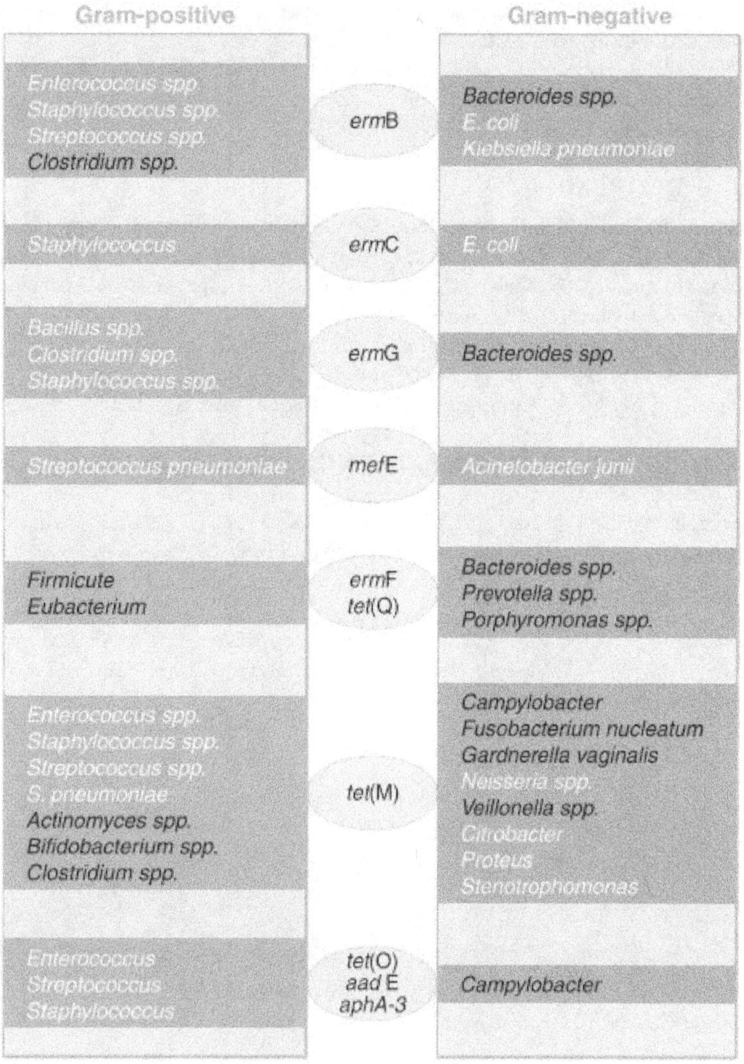

Evidence for transfer of resistance genes between gram-positive and gram-negative commensal bacteria and between aerobic (white typeface) and anaerobic (black typeface) species. This indirect evidence derives from the finding of virtually identical resistance genes (ovals) in the different species (blocks) isolated from the mammalian colon and from other environmental sites (not a complete listing). The resistances encoded are as follows: *erm, mef* = macrolides; tet = tetracyclines; aad, *aphA-3* = aminoglycosides. (Adapted from: A. Salyers et al., Trends Microbiol. **12**:412- 416, 2004; P. Courvalin, Antimicrob. Agents Chemother. **38**:1447–1451, 1994; K. K. Ojo et al., J. Antimicrob Chemother. **57**:1065–1069, 2006).

ACKNOWLEDGMENTS

This article is based on a meeting, coordinated by APUA, held in Boston on 2 June 2008 and supported by the National Biodefense Analysis and Countermeasures Center (NBACC) and the National Institute of Allergy and Infectious Disease through R24 grant AI50139.

Opinions, interpretations, conclusions, and recommendations are those of the authors and are not necessarily endorsed by the National Biodefense Analysis and Countermeasures Center (NBACC), Department of Homeland Security (DHS), or Battelle National Biodefense Institute (BNBI).

SUGGESTED READING

Alekshun M. N., and S. B. Levy. 2006. Commensals upon us. Biochem. Pharm. 71:893–900.

Andremont, A. 2003. Commensal flora may play key role in spreading antibiotic resistance. ASM News 69:601–607.

Barza, M., and S. L. Gorbach (ed.). 2002. The need to improve antimicrobial use in agriculture: ecological and human health consequences. Clin. Inf. Dis. Suppl. 3.

Blake, D. 2003. Transfer of antibiotic resistance between commensal and pathogenic members of the *Enterobacteriaceae* under ileal conditions. J. Appl. Microbiol. 95:428–436.

Dantas, G., M. O. A. Sommer, R. D. Oluwasegun, and G. M. Church. 2008. Bacteria subsisting on antibiotics. Science 320:100–103.

D'Costa, V. M., K. M. McGrann, D. W. Hughes, and G. D. Wright. 2006. Sampling the antibiotic resistome. Science 311:374–377.

Hummell, R., H. Tschape, and W. Witte. 1986. Spread of plasmid-mediated nourseothricin resistance in connection with antibiotic use in animal husbandry. J. Basic Microbiol. 26:461–466.

Levy, S. B. 2002. The antibiotic paradox: how the misuse of antibiotics destroys their curative powers, 2nd ed. Plenum Press, New York.

Martinez, J. L. 2008. Antibiotic and antibiotic resistance genes in natural environments Science 321:365–367.

White, D. G., M. N. Alekshun, and P. F. McDermott (ed.). 2005. Frontiers in antimicrobial resistance: a tribute to Stuart Levy. ASM Press, Washington, D.C.

Appendix 6: Zika: CDC Draft Interim Response Plan

Table of Contents

"The purpose of this document is to describe the Centers for Disease Control and Prevention (CDC) response plan for the first locally acquired cases of Zika virus infection in the continental United States and Hawaii. The Zika virus is spread to people primarily through the bite of an infected *Aedes aegypti* or *Aedes albopictus* mosquito. The response activities outlined in this plan are based on currently available knowledge about Zika virus and its transmission, and these activities may change as more is learned about Zika virus infection. Most of the plan focuses on response activities that would occur after locally acquired Zika virus transmission has been identified. CDC also is committed to responding to travel-associated and sexually transmitted Zika virus infections reported in the United States (US) before detection of the first locally transmitted case of Zika virus infection." (Centers for Disease Control and Prevention 2016b)